Narzulloyeva Dildora Saidjanovna

# DIAGNOSIS AND TREATMENT ALGORITHM FOR PATIENTS WITH CHRONIC HEART FAILURE

Monograph

© Narzulloyeva Dildora Saidjanovna
**Diagnosis and Treatment algorithm for patients with Chronic Heart failure**
By: Narzulloyeva Dildora Saidjanovna
Edition: January '2025
Publisher:
*Taemeer Publications LLC* (Michigan, USA / Hyderabad, India)

© **Narzulloyeva Dildora Saidjanovna**

| | | |
|---|---|---|
| Book | : | Diagnosis and Treatment algorithm for patients with Chronic Heart failure |
| Author | : | Narzulloyeva Dildora Saidjanovna |
| Publisher | : | Taemeer Publications |
| Year | : | '2025 |
| Pages | : | 110 |
| Title Design | : | *Taemeer Web Design* |

**BUKHARA – 2024**

**Narzulloyeva Dildora Saidjanovna** — Bukhara State Medical Institute, assistent of the department of faculty and hospital therapy, PhD.

**Reviewers:**

**1. Abdullaev R.B.** - TTA, Urgench branch, professor of Internal Medicine, reobiliotology and folk medicine, doctor of Medical Sciences

**2. Babajanova Z.X.**- Bukhara State Medical Institute Associate Professor of the Department of Propedeutics of Internal Diseases, PhD.

**Abstract:**

The pathological processes leading to CHF are numerous, among which coronary heart disease is the most widespread. There are several types of coronary heart disease, and in almost all cases, it can be complicated by CHF. Several factors are involved, including: the sympathoadrenal system, the renin-angiotensin-aldosterone system, the systolic and diastolic function of the heart, the catecholamine system, the humoral system, renal functional activity, and several other factors and systems are closely related. Among these, the functional state of the cardiovascular system plays a very important role in the pathogenesis of CHF. Although several studies have been conducted considering the functional state of the cardiovascular system, none have developed a clear algorithm for optimizing the treatment of patients suffering from chronic heart failure while taking into account the functional state of the cardiovascular system. This indicates the high relevance of this topic.

**Аннотация:**

СЮЕ га олиб келадиган патологик жараёнлар бир қанча бўлиб, улардан энг кенг тарқалгани юрак ишемик касаллиги ҳисобланади. Юрак ишемик касаллигининг бир қанча турлари мавжуд бўлиб, деярли барча ҳолатда СЮЕ билан асоратланиши мумкин. Бунда бир қанча омиллар, жумладан: симпатоадренал тизим, ренин ангиотензин альдостерин тизими, юракнинг систолик ҳамда диастолик фаолияти, катехоламин тизими, гуморал тизим, буйрак функционал фаолияти ва бошқа бир қанча омил ва тизимлар фаолиятига чамбарчас боғлиқ. Булар орасидан юрак қон томир функционал ҳолати СЮЕ патогенезида жудаям муҳим рол ўйнайди. Гарчи, юрак қон томир функционал ҳолатини инобатга олиб бир қанча тадқиқотлар ўтказилган бўлсада, уларнинг ҳеч бирида юрак қон томир функционал ҳолатини ҳисобга олган ҳолатда сурункали юрак етишмовчилиги билан оғриган беморларни даволашни отималлаштириш бўйича аниқ алгоритм ишлаб чиқилмаган. Бу эса ушбу мавзунинг жудям долзарблигидан далотат беради.

**Аннотация:**

Патологических процессов, приводящих к ХСН, существует несколько, наиболее распространенным из которых является ишемическая болезнь сердца. Существует несколько типов ишемической болезни сердца, и почти во всех случаях она может быть осложнена ХСН. При этом он тесно связан с несколькими факторами и системами, включая: симпатоадреналовую систему, ренин-ангиотензин-альдостериновую систему, систолическую и диастолическую функцию сердца, катехоламиновую систему, гуморальную систему, функциональную функцию почек и многие другие. Среди них очень важную роль в патогенезе ХСН играет сосудистое состояние сердца. Хотя было проведено несколько исследований с учетом функционального состояния сосудов сердца, ни в одном из них не был разработан точный алгоритм для оптимизации лечения пациентов с хронической сердечной недостаточностью с учетом функционального состояния сосудов сердца.

## 1. Chronic heart failure, its epidemiology and prevalence

Chronic heart failure (CHF) is a widely prevalent clinical syndrome that poses a significant burden on healthcare systems worldwide. Currently, 1-2% of the adult population in developed countries and 10% of the population over the age of 70 are suffering from CHF (Srisuk N, Cameron J, Ski CF, et al. Randomized controlled trial of family-based education for patients with heart failure and their carers. J Adv Nurs 2017). CHF is a disease that progresses and weakens patients, leading to a decrease in their quality of life and an increase in healthcare-related economic costs. CHF is a complex disease, and its diagnosis is determined by the physician based on the results of physical examinations, the patient's complaints, and the medical history (Ramani GV, Uber PA, Mehra MR. 2010). It is characterized by the heart's inability to meet the oxygen demands of peripheral cells and CHFC, as well as its negative impact on all organs (Tzanis G, Dimopoulos S, Agapitou V, Nanas S. 2014). The quality of life decreases in patients suffering from CHF, many patients experience a reduction in life expectancy, and the mortality rate within five years after diagnosis is high (Siabani S, Driscoll T, Davidson PM, Leeder SR. 2014). According to recent data, 5.8 million people in the United States suffer from chronic heart failure, while this figure reaches 23 million worldwide. In the United States, healthcare costs related to CHF amounted to $20.9 billion in 2012, and this figure is expected to reach $53.1 billion by 2030. However, considering the achievements in the medical treatment of cardiovascular diseases, the average life expectancy of the population is increasing, and it is anticipated that the number of patients suffering from CHF will rise in the coming years (Gaggin HK, Januzzi JL Jr. 2013). Considering the reforms and results being implemented in healthcare in the Republic of Uzbekistan,
it is undoubtedly true that the number of patients suffering from this pathological process will increase in the near future.

CHF is the leading cause of hospitalization in elderly patients. More than half of patients hospitalized with acute decompensation of heart failure are people older than 75 years, and about 20% are very old patients, that is, older than 85 years (Ramani GV, Uber PA, Mehra MR. 2010). The average age of patients with heart failure in different countries is different. This is probably related to lifestyle, food culture, life expectancy, health care system and social and economic factors in different countries. The average age of heart failure patients in Poland is 69.1±12.3 years (Polish ESC-HF Long Term Registry), and in the USA it is 73.2±14 years (OPTIMIZE-HF), and in Japan it is 72.9±13, 8 years old (ATTEND). Optimizing the management of heart failure in the elderly is a growing priority for the health care system, as the incidence of HF increases with the aging of the population, and the associated mortality and economic costs increase.

In our country, comprehensive work is being carried out to provide high-quality specialized cardiology medical care to the population and to implement high-tech methods of treatment. In 2017-2021, in accordance with the Action Strategy on the five priority directions of the development of the Republic of Uzbekistan, the important tasks of "improving the quality of medical and social-medical services, ensuring the reduction of morbidity rates among the population and prolongation of life" are defined in raising the level of medical services to the population to a new level. In the performance of these tasks, development of measures for the prevention of death and disability in health care centers and their application to other links of health care is considered one of the urgent directions.[1]

In order to further develop health care in the Republic of Uzbekistan, the task is to increase the quality of medical care in accordance with the development strategy for 2022-2026. Decree of the President of the Republic of Uzbekistan dated January 28, 2021 "On the new development strategy of Uzbekistan for 2022-2026" No. PF-60, 2021 No. PK-5199 of September 27 "On further development of the system of specialized medical care in the health sector the decision on improvement measures" and the decision of January 26, 2022 No. PQ-103 "On measures to improve the quality of prevention and treatment of cardiovascular diseases" as well as to implement the tasks specified in other regulatory and legal documents related to this activity this dissertation research serves a certain level.

---

[1] Decree of the President of the Republic of Uzbekistan dated February 7, 2017 No. PF-4947 "On the Strategy of Actions for the Further Development of the Republic of Uzbekistan"

Optimizing the effectiveness of treatment in patients with chronic heart failure, improving the quality of life of patients, increasing life expectancy, and reducing the length of stay in the hospital is an urgent problem of modern cardiology (Pfeffer MA, et al 2019, Metra M., 2021).

Despite the progress achieved in medicine, the single criteria for the treatment of patients with CHF have not yet been determined. Although many foreign researchers are working in this direction (Solomon S., 2022; McDonagh TA, 2021), there are enough problems waiting to be solved.

In recent years, research on the use of angiotensin-receptor-neprilysin-inhibitors in the treatment of patients with CHF is paying off (Greenberg B., 2020; Volpe M., 2019). Several studies have shown that this group of drugs improves the functional status of patients with heart failure with reduced ejection fraction and has a positive effect on central hemodynamic indicators (Niemiec R., 2022). Although the use of these drugs in clinical practice has not been long, the progress made indicates that these drugs are promising (PARADIGM-HF -study 2014y).

In addition to deterioration of the functional state, significant changes in the reserve volume of myocardial coronary vessels are also observed in patients with ischemic etiological CHF (Srivaratharajah K., 2016; Obokata M., 2018). In this case, sleep paralysis and hibernating myocardial CHF are of great importance. In this regard, optimization of treatment methods for patients suffering from CHF, study of effect of ARNI agents on reserve volume of coronary arteries and hibernating myocardium CHF, and optimization of therapeutic agents are undoubtedly considered urgent problems.

In our country, leading scientists such as Kurbonov R.D., Gadoev A.G., Abdullaev T.A., Kamilova U.K. have conducted scientific research on the problem of CHF. The role of neurohumoral, endothelial dysfunction and genetic factors in the outcome and course of CHF has been studied (Kurbonov R.D., 2016, Kamilova U.K., 2016). However, the effect of sacubitril/valsartan combination on the volume of coronary vessels and myocardial reserve in the treatment of patients with CHF of ischemic etiology has not been investigated in foreign and domestic studies conducted so far. This, in turn, requires the need to continue research in this direction.

Despite the progress achieved in the treatment of cardiovascular diseases (CVD), cardiovascular diseases remain the main cause of death in many countries of the world. The majority of patients over the age of 65 are patients with cardiovascular diseases, and 38 million people worldwide suffer from these diseases [8, p.35-48; 11, p. 812-824]. In 2017 alone, 17.8 million people died from STDs. This is 1/3 of all deaths in the world [7, 254-289; 12,]. According to the last annual report of the American Heart Association (American Heart Association), in 2016, 48% of older people have CVD [9, 13, p. 56-528]. Early detection and treatment of cardiovascular diseases can prevent premature death from cardiovascular diseases and increase the risk of developing heart failure (HF).

Cardiovascular diseases, including chronic heart failure (CHF), are pathological conditions that develop as a result of the influence of several genomic, genetic, environmental factors and lifestyle factors [8, p-344-379; 14, p. 142-146]. Year by year increase of CHF, cardiovascular diseases leading to this pathological process, i.e. ischemic heart disease and hypertensive diseases are among the most pressing isCHFC of modern medicine. Because the poor prognosis and high mortality rates pose a serious threat to human life and lead to increased economic costs for society and patients.

CHF is one of the main causes of death and disability in the world, and according to the definition of the American Heart Association and the American College of Cardiology, it is a complex clinical syndrome that leads to functional and structural disorders of the heart as a result of impaired contractility and relaxation of the ventricles. . According to the definition of the European Association of Cardiology, CHF is characterized by typical symptoms (shortness of breath, swelling of the ankles and fatigue) that can be observed with signs such as increased jugular vein pressure caused by structural and/or functional disorders of the heart, moist rales characteristic of heart failure in the lungs, and peripheral edema. is a characteristic clinical syndrome that causes a decrease in heart contraction activity and an increase in the pressure of the inner part of the heart at rest and during physical activity [7, p.15-67.]. According to the definition of Mentz and O'Connor, heart failure occurs as a result of dysfunction of the endothelium, kidney function, and venous system, resulting in remodeling of the myocardial structure, which in turn causes heart failure [6, p.23-82; 16, c. 28-35]. 5% of CVD cases correspond to heart failure. Currently, 26 million people worldwide suffer from heart failure. Of this, 6 million is the share of the USA, 15 million is the share of European countries [5, p.223-215; 17, p. 7-11]. CHF is a pathological process that is often preventable and leads to bad consequences if not treated in time. On average, 44% of patients with CHF are readmitted for cardiac or non-cardiac related conditions within 1 year of hospital discharge and receive an average of 4-6 days of inpatient care. In addition, it is observed that approximately half of the patients who are re-hospitalized have a delicate period within the first 12 weeks after the inpatient treatment (weakening of patients, exhaustion and increased likelihood of getting diseases) [3, p.79-80; 18, c. 1169-1186]. According to the results of a retrospective study, the rate of death from YuE decreased from 100 per 100,000 population in 1987 to 50 per 100,000 population in 2008, but at the same time, hospitalization related to CHF is increasing [7, p. 67-91; 19, p. 1-10].

Heart failure can be acute or chronic. CHF is considered a relatively stable process. Nevertheless, acute periods, i.e. decompensation processes, are observed in chronic heart failure. Chronic heart failure is often classified according to the New York Heart Association (NYHA) classification, which is evaluated by the severity of symptoms, their impact on the patient's physical activity and daily activities [8, 631-652; 19, p. 385-392]. Acute heart failure (AFF) is characterized by sudden worsening or rapid reappearance of clinical signs and symptoms of heart failure. Often AHF develops in patients with chronic heart failure as a result of aggravation of the disease, i.e. acute decompensation [7, p.56-78; 20, p. 385-392]. Heart failure can be divided into the following groups depending on the contractile activity of the myocardium: heart failure with reduced ejection fraction (EFCHF), in which the ejection fraction is less than ≤40%, heart failure with preserved ejection fraction

(OFCHF), in which the ejection fraction is greater than ≥50%, and ejection fraction is average reduced or borderline heart failure (EFCHF), in which the heart the firing fraction is in the range of 41%-49% [6, p.56-87; 21, p. 320-324].

Despite the advances in medicine and the discovery of new modern treatment and diagnosis methods, CHF remains a serious problem. Currently, 64 million people worldwide suffer from CHF. About half of them are patients with CHF with reduced ejection fraction. CHF is a chronic progressive disease, and approximately 50% of patients with this pathological process die within the next 5 years [4, 345-348; 22, p. 1121-1259]. If we look at the global statistics of diseases (Global Burden of Disease Studies), we can see that heart failure is a growing global epidemic and 17 million people are diagnosed with this disease per year [2, p.60-61; 23, pp. 117-171]. If we focus on the epidemiology of CHF, approximately half of this disease is CHF patients with reduced firing fraction. According to studies, the incidence rate of CHF is increasing and is expected to increase by approximately 46% by 2030. At the same time, it is predicted that the expenses related to CHF will increase in parallel [3, p.77; 24, p. 146-603].

It can be seen that there are differences in the mortality rate and the prevalence of this disease in patients with CHF across countries and regions. A recently published multi-country cohort study, INTER-CHF, showed a mortality rate of 16.5-7% in the People's Republic of China, 9% in South Africa and the Middle East, and 34% in African countries [ 8, pp. 633-634; 25, p. 665-672]. It can be observed that the 1-year death rate from CHF (13.6%) is higher in the countries of the southern region of Asia than in the countries of the northern part (8.9%). It can be seen that Indonesia (21.4%) and the Philippines (14.3%) are the countries with the highest 1-year mortality rate from CHF. On the other hand, although the majority of the population of Japan is elderly, it has been shown that the 1-year mortality rate from CHF is 4.4% [9, p.4-6; 26, pp.]. If we look at studies conducted in other countries, the incidence rate of CHF in the People's Republic of China is 1.3%, which indicates that 13.7 million of the population of this country are currently affected. 23% of them are heart failure with preserved ejection fraction (OFCHF), 23% are heart failure with moderately reduced ejection fraction (EFCHF), and 54% are heart failure with reduced ejection fraction (EFCHF) [4, 375-376; 27, p. 1329-1337]. If we focus on the statistical situation in the United States of America, 6.2 million residents of this country suffer from CHF, and this figure is bound to increase every year. In the United States, 915,000 new cases of heart failure occur each year. According to Gedela M. and his colleagues, the increase in the incidence rate of CHF is the result of an increase in the age group of the population, an increase in risk factors, an increase in the rate of recovery from acute coronary syndrome, and better treatment of other chronic diseases [10, p.35-36; 28, p. 403-405]. It has been shown that the annual increase in mortality and morbidity rates from CHF leads to an increase in the financial costs associated with this pathological process [29, p. 857-865]. The incidence rate of CHF is 20 cases per 1000 population under the age of 60-65, and 80 cases per 1000 population over the age of 80. Especially black Americans have been found to have a high risk of developing CHF [28, p. 403-405]. In the United States, the risk of developing CHF in people over 40 years of age has been shown to be 20%. In the statement of the European Association of Cardiologists, the prevalence of CHF among the population is 1-2%, and in the age group over 70 years it is higher than 10% [20, p. 385-392]. The risk of developing CHF in men over 55 years of age is 33%, and in women 28% [30, p. 891-975]. According to the results of a 10-year study on the epidemiology of CHF in the Russian Federation (EPOXA-XSN and EPOXA-O-XSN), it was shown that the prevalence of CHF in the western part of this country is 12.3%, and CHF in severe form is 2.3%.In the Russian Federation, the average death rate from CHF is 6%, that is, 612,000 people die from CHF and related complications in 1 year [7, p.9-14; 31, p. 7-77].

Hospital costs associated with CHF exceed $30 billion per year. The majority of these costs are related to hospital stays and return visits. Much of the research on the prevalence and incidence of heart failure is now being done in developed Western countries. According to a recent worldwide population-based study, the long-term prognosis of patients with CHF is strongly related to population location, gender, place of diagnosis, and socioeconomic status. From this, the authors concluded that it is more important to carry out treatment tactics adapted to each condition [32, p. 406-420].

As can be seen from the above facts, the incidence of CHF is increasing, and it is inextricably linked with the increasing age of the population, hypertension, chronic ischemic heart disease, obesity, hyperlipidemia, and diabetes. Most of the studies related to CHF have been conducted in the USA and European countries, and conducting research covering the epidemiology, risk factors, clinical course and economic costs of CHF in other parts of the world, including Uzbekistan, is considered one of the current isCHFC.

## 1.2. Clinical presentation and classification of chronic heart failure

*Clinical observations.* The most common clinical symptoms of CHF include shortness of breath, ankle or leg swelling, and fatigue. Although these symptoms are not inevitable, their presence indicates that patients should undergo further investigations to confirm the diagnosis. Although the causes and clinical course of left ventricular failure and right ventricular failure are similar, symptoms such as fatigue and shortness of breath in heart failure with left ventricular failure, peripheral edema and increased pressure in the spinal vein are more common in heart failure with right ventricular failure [22, c.1211–1259]. Due to compensatory mechanisms, early stages of heart failure may not have any obvious signs and symptoms. But as the disease progresses, the following signs and symptoms appear: tachycardia (sensitivity 7%, specificity 99%), leg swelling (sensitivity 10%, specificity 93%), dilatation of jugular veins (sensitivity 39%, specificity 92%), abnormal lung sounds ( wet wheezing) (sensitivity 60%, specificity 99%) is manifested to one degree or another [36, c.1981–1995]. Table 1 details the likelihood of experiencing signs and symptoms of heart failure (Table 1). Patients who have signs and symptoms of heart failure and these symptoms have not changed for at least 1 month are called stable CHF [37, c. 137–161]. In patients with stable CHF, it is called decompensated heart failure when their condition worsens. Table 2 lists the factors that lead to heart failure decompensation (Table 2). The classification of the New York Heart Association expresses the severity of symptoms and functional status in heart failure, while the Killip classification evaluates the severity of patients after acute myocardial infarction [37, c. 137–161].

**1 table.**

### Signs and symptoms of heart failure.

|  |  | Sensitivity (%) | Specificity (%) | Alternative causes |
|---|---|---|---|---|
| **Symptoms** | Panting | 66 | 52 | Respiratory diseases, anemia, obesity, fear |
|  | Paroxysmal nocturnal | 33 | 76 | Asthma, sleep apnea syndrome |

|  |  |  |  |  |
|---|---|---|---|---|
|  | panting |  |  |  |
|  | Orthopnea | 21 | 81 | Fear, obesity |
|  | The presence of swelling | 23 | 80 | Venous insufficiency, hypoproteinemia, drugs, hypoactivity, pneumonia, aspiration pneumonitis, sepsis, liver disease, kidney disease |
| Signs | Increased pressure in jugular veins | 10 | 97 | Pulmonary embolism, superior vena cava obstruction, pericardial fluid accumulation |
|  | 3 heart tones | 31 | 95 | Mitral regurgitation, fever, pregnancy |
|  | Peripheral tumors | 10 | 93 | Venous insufficiency, hypoproteinemia, drugs, inactivity |
|  | Tachycardia | 7 | 99 | Arrhythmias, pain, anxiety, fever, hypertension, drugs |
|  | Crepitation | 13 | 91 | Pulmonary fibrosis, chronic obstructive pulmonary disease, pneumonia, lung abscess, brochoectasis, bronchiolitis |

**2 tables.**

**Factors causing decompensation of heart failure.**

| Acute aggravators | Gradual aggravators |
|---|---|
| Acute coronary syndrome | Infections |
| Pulmonary artery embolism | Kidney dysfunction |
| Arrhythmias | Exacerbation of asthma or chronic obstructive pulmonary disease |
| Hypertensive crisis | Arrhythmias |
| Cardiac tamponade | Uncontrolled arterial hypertension |
| Aortic dissection | Anemia |
| Surgical complications | Hyperthyroidism or hypothyroidism |
| Peripartum cardiomyopathy | Non-adherence to treatment |

## 1.3. Modern pathophysiological mechanisms of development of chronic heart failure

***Cell mechanism.*** Unlike other cells in the human body, heart muscle cells, cardiomyocytes, do not reproduce by division. When a person is born, there are about 6 million cardiomyocytes, and these cells do not multiply during a person's life [43, c. 150-166]. However, cardiomyocytes may increase in size. In cardiomyocytes, this process is carried out by sarcomerogenesis, i.e. the creation and redistribution of new sarcomeres [44, c. 101-106]. Sarcomeres are functional contractile parts of heart cells, 1.7-2.1 µm long and consist of thick myosin and thin actin filaments [45, c. 641-651]. About 50 sarcomeres form a myofibril, and 50-100 myofibrils form a cardiomyocyte [46, c. 103-105]. Healthy cardiomyocytes are cylindrical, 80-100 µm long and 10-25 µm in diameter [47, c. 3-700].

***Excitability-contractility disorder.*** As mentioned above, chronic heart failure is divided into types with reduced ejection fraction (EFCHF) and preserved ejection fraction (OFCHF) depending on the ejection fraction. Disruption of the connection between excitability and contractility also plays an important role in the development mechanisms of EFCHF and OFCHF. Disturbance of excitability-contractility is often observed as a result of changes in cell membrane architecture, disruption of activity and production of $Ca^{2+}$-binding proteins, and inappropriate redistribution of intracellular $Ca^{2+}$ ions. These remodeling processes lead to a wide variety of transcriptional, conduction, metabolic, and electrophysiological changes. Finally, it causes the death of cardiomyocytes, which is observed in various forms of heart failure.

***Immune mechanisms in CHF.*** The presence of a constant inflammatory process in the body and, as a result, a high level of pro-inflammatory cytokines negatively affects the long-term remodeling of the ventricles [56, c. 1597-1600].

As a result of the mechanical stress of the left ventricle, inflammatory processes are activated in the myocardial CHF, leukocyte accumulation is observed, and the secretion of pro-inflammatory cytokines increases. Accumulation of macrophages leads to the development of hypertrophy, remodeling of the heart, formation of fibrotic CHF and reduction of left ventricular function.

***Importance of adrenergic nervous system in heart failure.*** Along with several systems, the adrenergic nervous system (ANS) plays an important role in the development of heart failure. If the heart function is normal, the activated ANS quickly returns to its place. If the changes in heart activity are chronic, even with the activation of ANS, the ability to maintain normal heart activity is lost, and chronic heart failure develops gradually.

## 1.4. Contemporary in chronic heart failure the importance of biomarkers

***Sodium uretic peptide system.*** The compensatory role of the sodium uretic peptide (SUP) system, which balances the overactivation of RAAS and ANS in CHF, has been known for 35 years. In the early stages of CHF, SUP stimulates diuresis, natriuresis, and vasodilation to reduce cardiac output and cardiac output. The concentration of SUP in plasma is inextricably linked with the weight of CHF [69, p. 223-241]. For this reason, SUP was accepted as a biomarker indicating the severity of the disease in CHF [70, p. 891-875]. Dysfunction of SUP is important in CHF syndrome, causing impaired water and sodium excretion, vasoconstriction, accumulation of fluid volume in the body, increased loading pressure, and deterioration of the patient's prognosis.

There are 3 types of sodium uretic peptide receptors in the body. They are: SUPR-A, SUPR-B and SUPR-S. SUPR-A and SUPR-B are guanylyl cyclase receptors, the activation of which increases the amount of cyclic guanosine monophosphate, which in turn increases the activity of downstream kinases [72, p. 419-425]. The interaction of SUP and its receptors has complex effects on the kidney, heart, blood vessels, endocrine system, cell growth and remodeling. In the heart, all three SUPs participate in anti-remodeling processes in the myocardium by controlling cell hypertrophy and collagen synthesis. In addition, SUP reduces the activity of RAAS (renin-angiotensin-aldosterone system) and SNS (sympathetic nervous system) and endothelin and arginine-vasopressin [73, p. 01-02].

***MicroRNA***(miRNA) is a non-coding ribonucleic acid of 22 nucleotides in size, which controls gene expression at the post-transcriptional level and plays an important role in the pathogenesis and progression of heart failure [14, p. 142-146].

***High sensitivity troponin.*** High-sensitivity cardiac troponin plays a unique biomarker role in cardiovascular diseases, including heart failure. Left ventricular dysfunction is more pronounced in patients with high levels of cardiac troponin. An increase in the amount of high-sensitivity cardiac troponin in CHF may be caused by a decrease in subendocardial perfusion as a result of the tension of the myocardial walls and a decrease in end-diastolic pressure.

***High-sensitivity S reactive protein.*** C reactive protein (CRP) is an acute phase proinflammatory cytokine produced in hepatocytes in response to the signal of interleukin-6 [77, p. 185-194]. The association of CRP with heart failure was first shown by Elster in 1956 [78, p. 185-194].

***Myeloperoxidase.*** Myeloperoxidase is an enzyme produced by leukocytes in response to inflammatory and oxidative stress processes, and can cause atherogenesis, rupture of atherosclerotic plaques, and remodeling of the left ventricle [84, p. 14766-14771].

***Growth-promoting soluble gene 2.*** Growth-promoting gene-2 (GPG 2) encodes protein expression for members of the interleukin-1 family (GPG 2L) and secretes soluble GPG 2, which is released from cardiac myocytes and fibroblasts in response to mechanical stretching of cardiac muscle [90, p. 827-840].

***Interleukin-6.*** Interleukin-6 is a proinflammatory cytokine that is synthesized by T lymphocytes against various stresses in the body, including heart failure [98, p. 643-651].

***Endothelin-1.*** Endothelin-1 is a vasoconstrictor produced by various cells.

***Galectin-3.*** Galectin-3 is a beta-galactoside related to the leptin family, which is produced in various organs, including myocardial CHF, in response to mechanical stress and inflammation.

## 1.5. Heart blood in chronic heart failure vascular functional status

***Reserve volume of coronary arteries in CHF with ischemic etiology***

When the coronary arteries are injured, the reserve volume of the coronary arteries or the expansion activity of the coronary microvascular vascular system is disturbed [113, p. 1782-1788]. If there is no narrowing of the coronary arteries, then the reserve volume of the coronary arteries is evaluated depending on the activity of the microvascular system. The reserve volume of coronary arteries is significantly reduced in several pathological conditions, such as arterial hypertension, obesity, and diabetes.

Resting coronary artery blood flow may be normal as long as 80-85% stenosis is observed. But the reserve volume of blood flow begins to decrease when the narrowing of the coronary arteries is 40-50%. The reserve volume of coronary arteries decreases by 2 times when the stenosis is 75%, and this indicates that ischemia is observed in the myocardium. Coronary artery reserve volume can be assessed by Doppler transthoracic echocardiography based on the difference in hyperemic blood flow at baseline and after drug-induced vasodilatation. First, the resting pressure of the left anterior descending artery is measured by Doppler signal, then adenosine is infused intravenously at a dose of 140 µg/kg/min, and after 1 minute the blood flow is re-evaluated by Doppler during diastole.

Transthoracic echocardiography is considered the gold standard in the diagnosis of chronic heart failure. Because through this examination, it is possible to fully assess the functional activity of the myocardium. With this, we can measure left ventricular contraction activity, ejection fraction, left ventricular and interventricular septal thickness, then diastolic volume, then diastolic pressure, then systolic volume, then systolic pressure, ejection fraction, cardiac output, left ventricular width, left ventricular cavity width. , right ventricular and right ventricular dimensions, and several other cardiac functional activities can be evaluated.

If we consider chronic heart failure as a mechanical dysfunction of the heart, it is important to evaluate the activity of the left ventricle at each contraction of the heart, which corresponds to a certain part of the end-diastolic volume of the left ventricle. For the first time, Folse and Braunwald used radioisotope methods to evaluate the activity of the left ventricle [117, p. 674-685]. Later, Bartle evaluated the function of the left ventricle by an angiographic method [118, p. 125] and thus the concept of left ventricular ejection fraction appeared. Currently, the main classification of heart failure is based on the reduction of the ejection fraction. The concept of sleep and hibernating myocardium first appeared in science in 1980 and attracted considerable attention. This phenomenon is observed in myocardial ischemia and is observed in many cases after myocardial infarction. In 1982, Braunwald and Kloner named the concept of myocardium paralysis as prolonged ventricular dysfunction after a period of nonlethal ischemia [122, p. 1149-1149]. They defined myocardial stiffness as a condition during acute ischemia and contractile dysfunction after prolonged ischemia. Taking into account that the hibernating myocardium is the myocardial cells that have not yet died, but do not continue to function, it is seen that the recovery of the activity of the hibernating myocardium is important in patients with CHF of ischemic etiology [123, p. 263-327]. Determining the reserve volume of the myocardium is important in assessing the vasomotor activity of the myocardium and microvascular dysfunction.

Decreased reserve of myocardial CHF leads to an increase in left ventricular filling pressure and a decrease in heart rate, which in turn causes symptoms of heart failure, such as shortness of breath, and an increase in mortality [130, p. 3293-3302]. In this case, the reserve volume of the myocardium decreases and the density of coronary microcircular vessels decreases [132, p. 550-559]. In heart failure with preserved and reduced ejection fraction, the increase in blood filling pressure of the left ventricle during physical activity, together with the structural and functional changes of the myocardium, endangers the blood flow in the myocardial CHF, which causes the development of subendocardial ischemia and damage to the heart cells. According to studies, it was observed that the systolic and diastolic reserve volume of the left ventricle was reduced in CHF [133, p. 2138-2147]. A decrease in the diastolic reserve volume causes an increase in the blood filling pressure of the left ventricle, as a result of which there is an increase in shortness of breath, the development of hypertension in the pulmonary artery, and an increase in mortality [134, p. 3103-3112].

## 1.6. In chronic heart failure
## block neurohumoral control systems

Neurohumoral mechanisms play an important role in the development of CHF. In particular, the importance of the sympatho-adrenal system and the renin-angiotensin-aldosterone system is incomparable.

***Sympathetic nervous system.*** The importance of the autonomic nervous system in controlling cardiovascular activity is incomparable. In particular, the decreased ABP in CHF reduces the excitation of carotid baroreceptors, as a result of which the influence of the sympathetic nervous system on the kidneys increases [137, p. 1913-1920].

SNS affects several organs, causing systemic vasoconstriction and increased venous vascular tone. Through this, it is possible to increase the preload of the heart and keep the number of heart contractions at a normal level for a certain period of time. Normally, norepinephrine released from sympathetic nerve nodes leads to contraction of afferent arterioles and a decrease in blood flow in the kidney [139, p. 41-48]. In CHF, the sensitivity of renal blood vessels to depolarization increases, but the sensitivity to α1 phenylephrine agonists and blunt α2 receptors remains unchanged [140, p. 429-437]. On the other hand, as a result of increased calcium permeability and sensitivity and increased nitric oxide release, the sensitivity of α1 receptors increases, as determined in several CHF models in systemic arteries [141, p. 393-401]. Norepinephrine increases tubular reabsorption in the proximal and distal parts. The increase in oxygen demand, which is observed as a result of increased reabsorption and decreased blood flow, leads to a decrease in oxygen saturation of the kidneys.

In systolic dysfunction, there is an increase in neurohormonal activity in order to maintain adequate heart contractions. The neuronal effect is manifested by the activation of the SNS and the decrease in the activity of the parasympathetic nervous system, and the humoral effect is manifested by the increase in the production of certain hormones, such as in the renin-angiotensin-aldosterone system. Increased activity of the sympathetic nervous system in CHF can lead to impaired left ventricular diastolic function, which is a specific risk for cardiovascular activity.

***Renin-angiotensin-aldosterone system.*** The importance of the renin-angiotensin-aldosterone (RAAS) system in the pathophysiology of CHF is immeasurable. The ability of this system to adapt to a rapidly changing environment when the ability of the vital organs to respond to the body's requirements is reduced indicates its high importance in the pathophysiology of CHF. RAAS is activated as a result of stimulation of the sympathetic nervous system and reduction of blood flow in the renal arteries. The most important product in this cascade reaction is angiotensin II, which has several properties and has a compensatory nature in the early stages, which leads to the worsening of the CHF syndrome as the disease progresses.

Sympathetic nervous system is also closely related to RAAS, excessive release of catecholamines as a result of their inotropic and chronotropic effect increases heart contractions for a certain period of time, but in later stages increases the risk of myocardial CHF ischemia, hypertrophy, and arrhythmia development [145, p. 187-189]. In contrast, the sodium uretic peptide system has an antagonistic effect on SNS and RAAS. In response to the stretching of the myocardial CHF wall as a result of the activation of SNS and RAAS, type A and type B sodium uretic peptides are synthesized and block the activity of counter mediators, leading to expansion of peripheral blood vessels and natriuresis. These peptides are partially degraded by the enzyme neprelysin, which is important in the treatment of CHF [146, p. 993-1004]. Although RAAS and SNS are generally positive in the initial stage of heart failure, as the disease progresses, they have an adverse effect on natriuresis and vasodilation, causing worsening of the heart failure syndrome.

Aldosterone, an end product of the renin-angiotensin-aldosterone system, plays an important role in the regulation of blood pressure, body fluid content, and electrolyte homeostasis. In addition, aldosterone, as a result of excessive activation of mineralocorticoid receptors, causes arterial hypertension, atherosclerosis, vascular injury, heart failure and chronic kidney diseases, as well as several other diseases associated with endothelial CHF dysfunction [147, p. 1243-1248]. Due to the importance of RAAS in cardiovascular diseases, arterial hypertension and kidney diseases, there is no doubt that the effectiveness of ACEII, ARB, MRA drugs in these diseases is huge.

***Natriuretic peptide.***The natriuretic peptide system plays an important role in the course of CHF by opposing renin-angiotensin-aldosterone and sympathetic nervous system activity in CHF. Activation of the natriuretic peptide system in the early stages of CHF causes increased diuresis, natriuresis, and vasodilation and reduces cardiac output and cardiac output. For this reason, in the early stages of CHF, the concentration of natriuretic peptide in plasma increases proportionally to the severity of CHF, in this regard, this biomarker can be used to assess the severity of the disease [149, p. 891-975]. But in the later stages of the disease, the effect of natriuretic peptide decreases and patients experience sodium retention, fluid retention, vasoconstriction, and increased pressure.

In addition to controlling extracellular fluid and blood pressure, SUP also controls several metabolic processes. There are at least 3 SUP receptors in the body: SUP-A, SUP-B and SUP-S. Among them, SUP-A and SUP-B are guanylcyclase receptors, their activation causes activation of cyclic guanosine monophosphate, which in turn causes activation of the kinase system [150, p. 321-328]. The interaction of SUP with receptors is manifested by complex processes of influence, such as renal, vascular, cardiac, endocrine activity, cell growth and CHF remodeling.

In the early stages of CHF, brain SUP and brain SUP play an important role in maintaining the balance of sodium and homeostasis in the body. However, as CHF progresses, the effect of SUP decreases and its natriuresis, vasodilation, and hormonal suppressive effects are impaired, resulting in increased sodium absorption, vascular vasoconstriction, which in turn accelerates CHF progression. As a result, the synthesis of SUP in the plasma increases and its concentration in the blood increases. The rise of CHF will cause the activities of SNS and RAAS to further surpass the SUP system.

## 1.7. Pharmacology of chronic heart failure modern approaches to treatment

Modern treatment principles of CHF are being optimized with the understanding of its pathophysiology and the development of new drugs. After 1980, CHF was recognized as a neurohormonal disorder, and physicians focused on blocking RAAS and SNS. ACEI inhibitors [152, p. 1575-1581] and beta-blockers have been shown in studies to improve contractility of the left ventricle [153, pp.

2807-2816]. Mineralocorticoid receptor antagonists have also been shown to be effective in patients with CHF when used together with ACEI inhibitors and beta blockers [154, pp. 48-57]. Angiotensin receptor blockers are also effective in patients with CHF with reduced ejection fraction, and are used as an alternative drug when ACEI inhibitors are contraindicated or develop side effects [155, p., 767-771].

Pharmacological drugs used taking into account neurohormonal activity significantly improved disease prognosis compared to inotropic and vasodilator drugs in patients with CHF with reduced firing fraction [156, p., 1030-1039].

By the 2000s, several other drugs were recommended for the treatment of CHF. One of them is ivabradine, which blocks if channels in the sinoatrial node, thereby reducing the number of heart contractions independently of beta blockers. In patients with CHF with reduced ejection fraction, ivabradine has been shown to improve clinical outcomes and prognosis in patients with a heart rate greater than 70 regardless of beta-blockers [157, pp. 875-888].

In 2014, the results of the PARADIGM-HF study were published and the effectiveness of a new group of drugs, angiotensin-receptor-neprilysin inhibitors (ARNI), in patients with CHF with reduced firing fraction was widely recognized [3, p.80-81; 149, pp. 993-1004]. ARNI is a combination of valsartan and sacubitril, a neprilysin inhibitor. Neprilysin is an endogenous enopeptidase, which is involved in the degradation of several endogenous vasoactive peptides, including bradykinin, adrenomodulin. By blocking neprilysin, sacubitril increases the concentration of these endogenous peptides, which counteracts the increase in neurohormonal activity. Studies have shown that when ARNIs and ACEIi are used together, neurohormonal activity is further reduced, which in turn alleviates the progression of CHF. According to the results of a randomized study, ARNI drugs reduce the rates of mortality and hospital readmissions in patients with CHF with reduced ejection fraction compared to ACEIIs. Currently, ARNI drugs are widely used in practice for the treatment of patients with CHF with reduced ejection fraction. The significance of this group of drugs in patients with CHF with preserved ejection fraction and myocardial infarction is now widely studied by scientists of the world community.

***New drugs.*** Sodium glucose cotransporter-2 (SGC-2) inhibitors and glucagon-like peptide antagonists. SGC-2 inhibitors are new antiglycemic drugs that increase urinary glucose excretion from renal tubules [1, 34-35; 160, p., 1643-1658]. According to the results of a large randomized study, empagliflozin showed effective results. Empagliflozin reduced rehospitalization and cardiovascular mortality in patients with type 2 diabetes, and no serious side effects other than urinary tract infections were observed (EMPA-REG OUTCOME study). Canagliflozin also reduced the risk of developing cardiovascular disease and death in patients with type 2 diabetes (CANVAS study). However, in the group receiving canafliglozin, the rate of bone fractures and amputation was higher than in the placebo group [5, p. 213-214; 160, pp. 644-657]. SGC-2 inhibitors increase glucosuria and diuresis, thereby reducing blood pressure, improving glycemic control, reducing body weight, and improving insulin resistance. Alternatively, SGC-2 inhibitors show a cardioprotective effect due to the improvement of cardiac metabolism. According to the results of a large randomized study, liraglutide, a glucagon-like peptide antagonist, has been shown to reduce cardiovascular disease and all types of mortality [2, p.63-64; 161, pp. 311-322]. But this group of drugs is currently undergoing research in order to evaluate their exact mechanisms and prove their effectiveness.

***Angiotensin-converting enzyme inhibitors (ACEIs).*** Angiotensin-converting enzyme inhibitors are one of the main drugs in the treatment of patients with CHF. ACEIs reduce clinical symptoms, mortality and rehospitalization in patients with CHF.

In 1987, the drug enalapril was tested for the first time in a patient with IV FC according to CHF NYHA and reduced the mortality rate by 27% (CONSENSUS Trial) [162, p. 1429-1435], and in patients with II-III FC according to NYHA, it reduced the mortality rate by 16% (SOLVD Trial) [163, p. 293-302]. In another study of low- and high-dose lisinopril in patients with heart failure with reduced NYHA ejection fraction II-IV FC, treatment with high-dose lisinopril reduced hospital admissions and mortality by 15% compared with low-dose lisinopril (ATLAS Trial). [164, p. 2312-2318]. According to the meta-analysis, the use of ACEIi after myocardial infarction, including enalapril, reduces the rate of hospitalization and death by 27% [152, p. 1575-1581].

According to studies, different ACEIIs have shown almost similar effectiveness in CHF. Contraindications to the use of drugs of this group are the presence of angineurotic edema in the anamnesis, pregnancy. Alternatively, these drugs should be used with caution when systolic blood pressure is low, when blood creatinine is high, when there is stenosis of both renal arteries, or when the potassium level in the blood is higher than 5 mmol/l. Treatment with ACEIIs is started in small doses and titrated by checking blood potassium and kidney function every 1-2 weeks.

Side effects associated with this group of drugs are closely related to angiotensin and kinase enzymes. Among the side effects, dry cough is observed in about 20% of patients. In rare cases, severe angioedema may occur. ACEI inhibitors have been shown to improve clinical symptoms in patients with preserved CHF ejection fraction, although they do not reduce mortality. However, in one study, treatment with perindopril reduced the number of cardiovascular events by 31% and the number of rehospital visits by 37% compared to the placebo group in patients older than 70 years with preserved ejection fraction (PEF-CHF Trial) [165, p., 2338 - 2345].

Thus, today, in order to prevent complications and improve the prognosis in the treatment of CHF, special importance is attached to the optimization of the treatment taking into account the functional state of the heart and blood vessels, the reserve volume of the myocardium and modern biomarkers. Considering that many researches aimed at the study of CHF continue in different directions and that this disease is comprehensive, it can be understood that there are many questions that are still waiting to be answered in this direction. In this regard, it can be concluded that modern treatment tactics are necessary in accordance with the cardiovascular continuum, myocardial functional status, and the amount of modern biomarkers in the treatment of patients with ischemic etiology who suffer from CHF. Additional studies are required to evaluate the effect and effectiveness of a drug or a combination of drugs in a specific pathological process.

## 2.1. Characterization of study patients according to left ventricular ejection fraction and disease phenotypic groups

### 2.1.1. Clinical demographic characteristics of patients

Patients with a reduced ejection fraction of chronic heart failure (EFCHF ≤40%) in the examination accounted for 45%, patients with an average ejection fraction 25% (AEFCHF 41-49%), and patients with preserved ejection fraction 30% (OFCHF ≥50%).

Patients with chronic heart failure with reduced ejection fraction were younger (mean age 66.4 ± 12.0 years), and men were more common than women (69.5%), in contrast to patients with slightly reduced ejection fraction and preserved ejection fraction. At the same time, the majority of patients in this group were smokers (30.0%). 82% of patients in this group had a history of myocardial infarction and underwent percutaneous intervention (stenting and balloon angioplasty) or aortic coronary bypass surgery, and the remaining 18% were patients suffering from chronic ischemic heart disease. 30% of patients with chronic heart failure with reduced ejection fraction have chronic kidney disease (non-terminal).

Most of the patients who were saved by the shooting fraction were older and elderly patients. The average age of patients with this phenotype was 74.2±11.6 years. The majority of patients of this category were women (71%) and arterial hypertension was often observed (84%). 25% of patients with preserved firing fraction had a history of various disorders of blood circulation in the brain. It was observed that 31% of patients had anemia of various degrees in their anamnesis. At the same time, the anamnesis of the patients of this contingent was less frequent of IKKS and percutaneous interventions compared to the patients with CHF with reduced ejection fraction (44%), but the frequency of suffering from chronic coronary syndrome was observed more (48%).

Patients with a moderate reduction in ejection fraction had an intermediate score between patients with reduced ejection fraction and patients with preserved ejection fraction. Among the patients in this contingent, 49% were men and 51%

were women. In this contingent, smokers were observed relatively less (11%). Arterial hypertension and coronary syndrome of chronic heart were more common in patients of this contingent (87% and 64%, respectively). 53% of patients had a history of myocardial infarction. 38% of patients were found to have heart rhythm disorders (including ventricular fibrillation). Patients with all phenotypes were characterized by a high degree of comorbidity according to Charlson. No differences were found in this category of patients with chronic obstructive pulmonary disease, diabetes and body weight index (Table 6).

**6 tables.**

**Clinical demographic parameters of patients with chronic heart failure according to ejection fraction**

| Indicator | EFCHF n=54 | AEFCHF n=30 | OFCCHF n=36 |
|---|---|---|---|
| Age, year | 66.4±12.0 | 69.5±11.8 | 74.2±11.6* |
| Gender male/female, n(%) | (69.5)/(30.5) | (49)/(51) | (71)/(29) |
| TMI, kg/m2 | 32.5±6.2 | 33.4±6.8 | 32.7±6.4 |
| Smoking, n(%) | 16 (30)** | 2 (6) | 4 (11) |
| Alcohol, n(%) | 3 (5) | 2 (7) | 1 (3) |
| Angina: FC - II FC - III FC – IV | 12(10) 20 (16.7) 22(18.3) | 10(8.3) 12(10) 8(6,7) | 14(11.7) 12(10) 10(8.3) |
| IKKS, n(%) | 44 (82)** | 30 (53)* | 10 (28) |
| Percutaneous coronary intervention, n(%) | 7 (13) | 3 (10) | 4 (11) |
| In US anamnesis, n(%) | 5 (10) | 2 (7) | 5 (14) |
| Arterial hypertension, n(%) | 49 (91) | 27 (90) | 33 (92) |
| Diabetes, n(%) | 26 (48) | 12 (40) | 11 (30) |
| Volatility constant form of | 18 (33) | 11 (38) | 12 (33) |

| fractions, n(%) | | | |
|---|---|---|---|
| Status after UNFCCC, n(%) | 7 (13) | 5 (17) | 9 (25) |
| SBK, n(%) | 16 (30) | 8 (27) | 8 (22) |
| Anemia, n(%) | 8 (15) | 7 (23) | 13 (36)* |
| OSOK, n(%) | 11 (20) | 8 (27) | 7 (19) |
| Charlson scale | 7 | 7 | 7 |

Note: *r<0.05, r**<0.01 – patients with decreased firing fraction compared to the phenotype;

### 2.1.2. Chronic heart failure provoking factors of decompensation

The analysis of patients with chronic heart failure showed that 22% of the total patients did not take medications on time and did not follow the doctor's recommendations. In addition, in 18% of patients, decompensation of chronic heart failure was observed as a result of heart rhythm disturbances, in which ventricular flutter played the main role (paroxysmal ventricular flutter in the majority of patients 68%, persistent ventricular flutter 27%, ventricular extrasystole 5%). Decompensation of chronic heart failure was caused by hypertensive crises in 12% of cases. Of these, 7% of patients noted that the crisis developed due to non-compliance with the recommended diet, and 5% of patients noted that the crisis developed due to excessive consumption of table salt.

It was found that 35% of decompensation of CHF occurred due to infectious inflammatory diseases of the respiratory system. In the remaining 13%, it was not possible to determine the cause of decompensation of CHF. In the following 3 pictures, the reasons for decompensation of CHF are given.

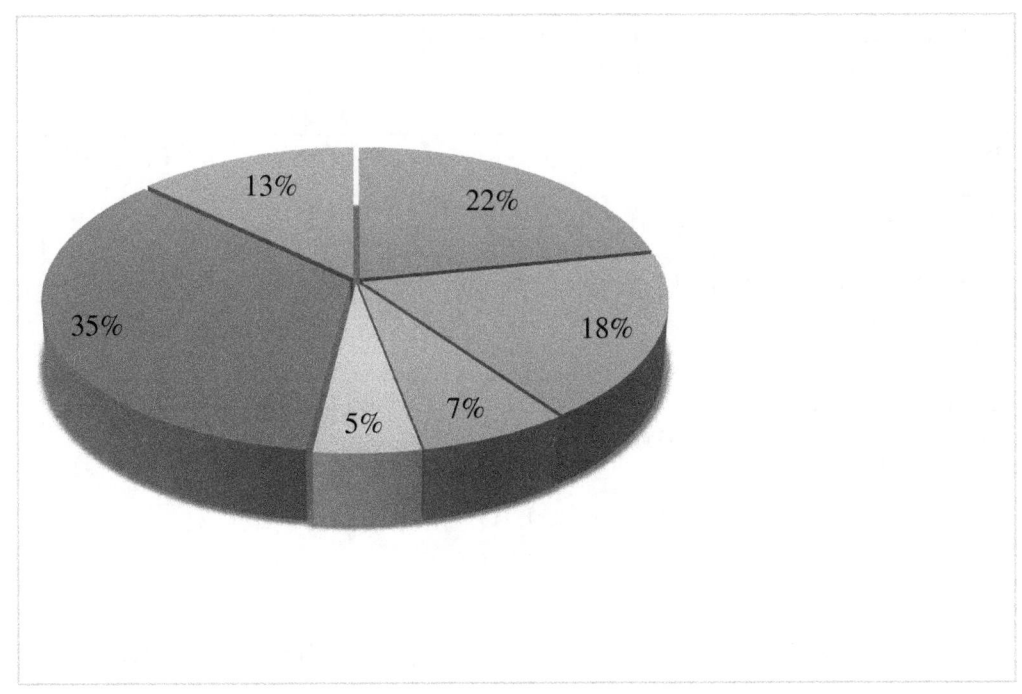

Note: Statistically significant difference when R < 0.05
**3 pictures. The main reasons for the decompensation of CHF.**

The main cause of decompensation in patients with chronic heart failure with reduced ejection fraction was the failure to take medication on time, followed by heart rhythm disorders and infectious diseases of the respiratory system. In patients with a slightly reduced ejection fraction, heart rhythm disturbances and infectious diseases of the respiratory organs were the main cause of decompensation. Instability of arterial blood pressure and diseases of respiratory organs were the main cause of decompensation of CHF in patients with preserved ejection fraction, followed by failure to take medication on time. At the same time, in 11% of these contingent patients, heart rhythm disturbances (paroxysmal form of ventricular flutter in 6, extrasystole in 1) caused decompensation of CHF (table 7).

**7 tables**

**The main reasons for the decompensation of CHF depending on the left ventricular ejection fraction**

| Reasons | EFCHF n=54 | AEFCHF n=30 | OFCCHF n=36 |
|---|---|---|---|
| | | | |

| | | | |
|---|---|---|---|
| Non-adherence to drug treatment recommendations, n (%) | 16 (30)* | 5 (17) | 4 (14) |
| Infectious diseases, n (%) | 10 (18) | 18 (60)*** | 14 (38) |
| Non-adherence to the diet, n (%) | 0 | 1 (3) | 7 (19)** |
| Excessive consumption of table salt, n (%) | 1 (2) | 1 (3) | 4 (11)* |
| Cardiac arrhythmias, n (%) | 11 (20) | 7 (23)* | 4 (11) |
| Unknown, n (%) | 7 (13) | 3 (10) | 3 (8) |

Note: (*$p<0.05$, **$p<0.01$, ***$p<0.001$) – firing fraction decreased compared to the patients phenotype

Thus, 40% of patients with chronic heart failure with reduced ejection fraction, 30% of patients with preserved ejection fraction, and 30% of patients with moderately reduced ejection fraction. Factors causing decompensation of CHF include infectious inflammatory diseases of respiratory organs (35%), non-compliance with medication recommendations (22%), heart rhythm disorders (18%) (paroxysmal ventricular flutter in most patients 68%, persistent ventricular flutter 27%, ventricular extrasystole 5 %), cases of hypertensive crisis (13%).

### 2.1.3. Clinical and hemodynamic parameters of patients included in the study according to ejection fraction.

In the examination, symptoms such as shortness of breath (89%; n=107), leg swelling (79%; n=95), fatigue (81%; n=97) were observed during physical activity. More than half of the patients had pulmonary edema, as assessed by small-bubble moist crackles on endoscopy in the lungs (59%; n=71) as well as evidence of pulmonary edema on X-ray examination (49%; n=59). Orthopnea was found in 38% (n=46) of examined patients. Hepatomegaly was found in 42% (n=50) patients (Table 8).

**8 tables**

**Clinical characteristics of patients with chronic heart failure according to left ventricular ejection fraction (n=120)**

| Indicator | General n=120 | EFCHF n=54 | AEFCHF n=30 | OFCCHF n=36 |
|---|---|---|---|---|
| Fatigue, n (%) | 97 (81%) | 50 (92%) | 21 (70%)* | 26 (72%)* |
| Wheezing at rest, n (%) | 57 (48%) | 39 (72%) | 12 (40%)** | 7 (19%)*** |
| Panting during physical exertion, n (%) | 107 (89%) | 51 (94%) | 27 (90%) | 29 (80.5%)* |
| Orthopnea, n (%) | 44 (37%) | 22 (41%) | 11 (37%)* | 11 (30%)* |
| Tumors, n (%) | 95 (79%) | 43 (79%) | 23 (77%) | 29 (81%) |
| Wheezing in the lungs, n (%) | 71 (59%) | 34 (63%) | 17 (56%)* | 20 (55%)* |
| Hepatomegaly, n (%) | 50 (42%) | 29 (53.7%) | 11 (37%)** | 10 (28%)*** |
| Signs of hemostasis according to X-ray examination, n(%) | 59 (49%) | 25 (46%) | 15 (50%) | 19 (53%)* |

Note: (*$p<0.05$, **$p<0.01$, ***$p<0.001$) – patients with decreased firing fraction compared to the phenotype;

In patients with chronic heart failure with reduced ejection fraction, clinical symptoms such as weakness (92%), shortness of breath at rest (72%), shortness of breath during physical activity (94%) prevailed among the general clinical complaints. Orthopnea was observed in 41% of patients, and hepatomegaly in 53.7% of patients.

Patients with chronic heart failure with preserved ejection fraction had more peripheral edema (81%) than patients with reduced ejection fraction and moderately reduced ejection fraction, and X-ray signs of hemostasis were found to be higher than other phenotypes (53%).

Patients with mildly reduced ejection fraction had clinical symptoms intermediate to those of patients with reduced ejection fraction and preserved ejection fraction CHF. 70% of patients with this phenotype had fatigue, 40% rested dyspnea, 90% exertional dyspnoea, 37% orthopnea, 77% edema, 56% wheezing, 37% hepatomegaly, and 46% X-ray examination of small signs of blood clotting were observed in the circulatory system. 81% of patients with reduced ejection fraction had

CHF III/IV FC, compared to 67% in patients with moderately reduced ejection fraction and 61% in OFCCHF patients (Fig. 4).

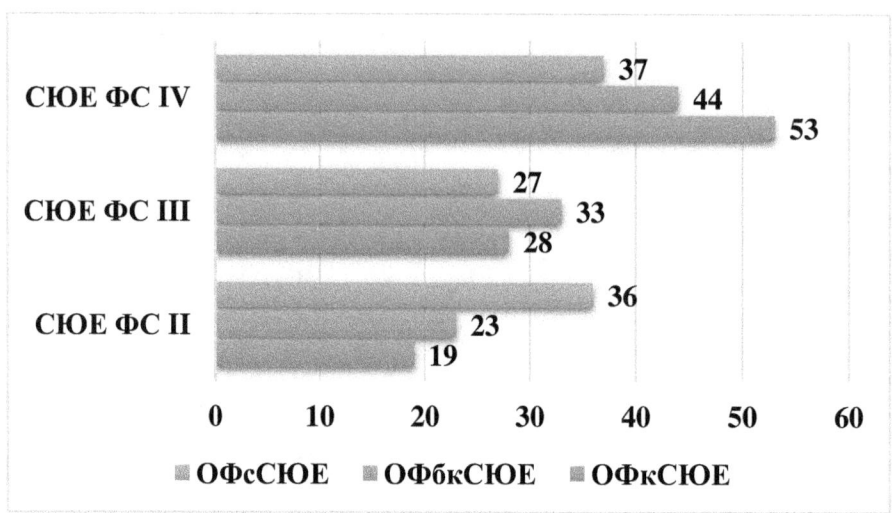

Note: Statistically significant difference when p < 0.05

**4 pictures. Distribution of functional classes among patients according to phenotypes of left ventricular ejection fraction in chronic heart failure (n=120).**

According to the results of a 6-minute test conducted on patients, the average distance traveled in patients with chronic heart failure with a reduced ejection fraction was 168.5±35.0 meters, in patients with an average reduced ejection fraction it was 234.2±56.0 meters, and in patients with a preserved ejection fraction it was 287. It was 3±62.5 meters. In addition, the minute oxygen consumption index was 11.4±4.6 ml/(kgxmin) in patients with EFCHF, 13.5±5.1 ml/(kgxmin) in patients with AEFCHF, and 14 in patients with OFCCHF. was 1±6.9 ml/(kgxmin) (Fig. 5).

When hemodynamic parameters of patients were analyzed, it was observed that patients with chronic heart failure with reduced ejection fraction had lower arterial blood pressure and higher number of heart contractions. In this case, the lowest indicator of HB was observed in the phenotype of patients with OFCCHF (Table 9).

**9 tables.**

**Variation of SAKB and DAKB and YUKS depending on the firing fraction**

| Indicators | EFCHF n=54 | AEFCHF n=30 | OFCCHF |
|---|---|---|---|

|  |  |  | n=36 |
|---|---|---|---|
| SABP, mm.sm.ust. | 129.6±19.2 | 132.4±21.4 | 142.7±30.6* |
| DABP, , mm.sm.ust. | 76.5±11.8 | 79.4±14.6 | 82.4±15.0* |
| Average ABP, mm.cm.asl. | 107.8±14.9 | 109.6±17.8 | 112.0±21.2* |
| HIGH, th/min | 95.4±22.0 | 87.4±26.4* | 84.6±24.0** |

Note: *r<0.05, r**<0.01 – patients with decreased firing fraction compared to the phenotype

In patients with chronic heart failure with reduced ejection fraction, systolic arterial blood pressure in the range of 100-140 mm Hg was more typical. It was observed that 90-110 beats/min is characteristic of patients with this phenotype. At this time, it was observed that systolic, diastolic and average blood pressure was higher in patients with OFCCHF than in patients with other phenotypes, and it was observed that systolic, diastolic and average blood pressure was characteristic of 70-90 beats/min (pictures 6, 7, 8).

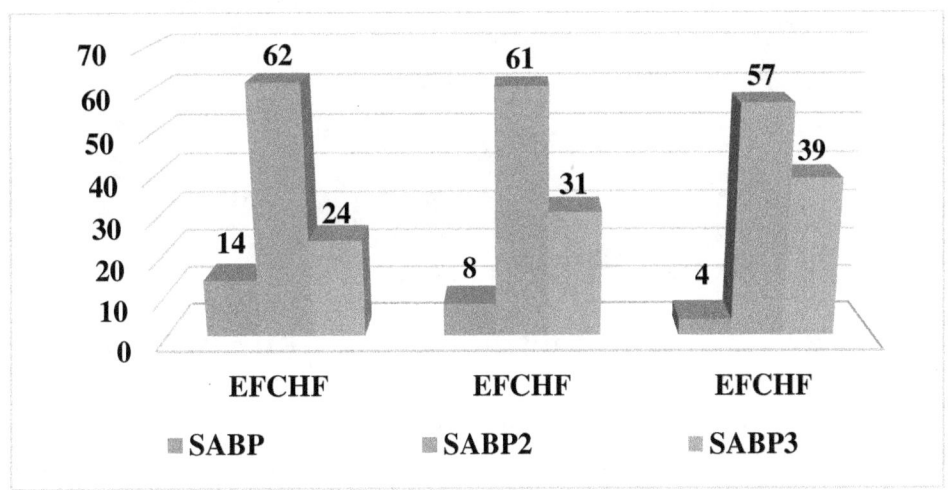

Note: Statistically significant difference when p < 0.05

**6 pictures. Value of patients' initial systolic arterial blood pressure (SABP) depending on the phenotypes of the left ventricular ejection fraction.**

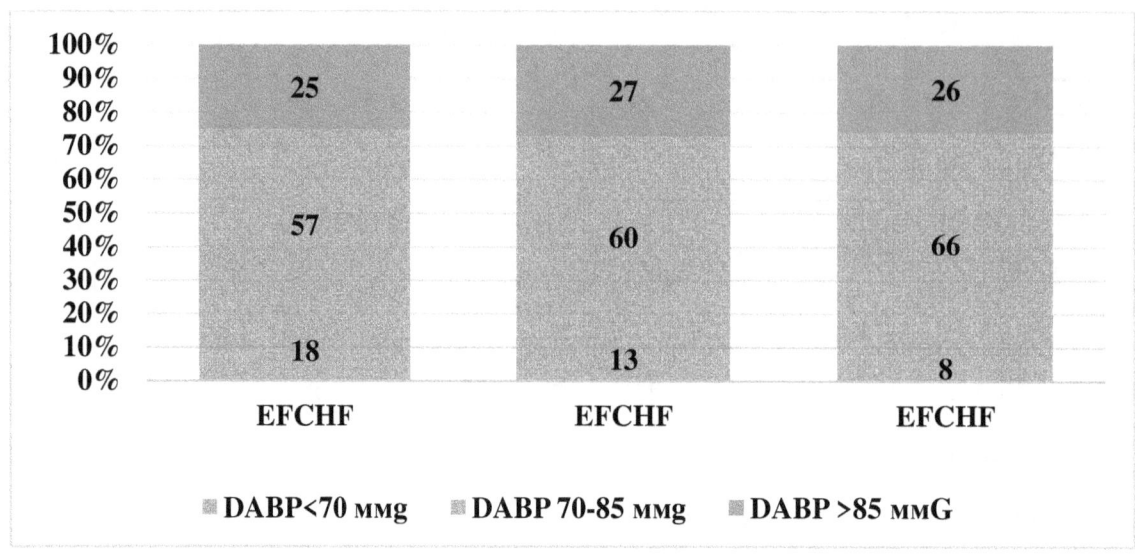

Note: Statistically significant difference when p < 0.05

**7 pictures. Value of initial diastolic arterial blood pressure (DABP) of patients according to phenotypes of left ventricular ejection fraction.**

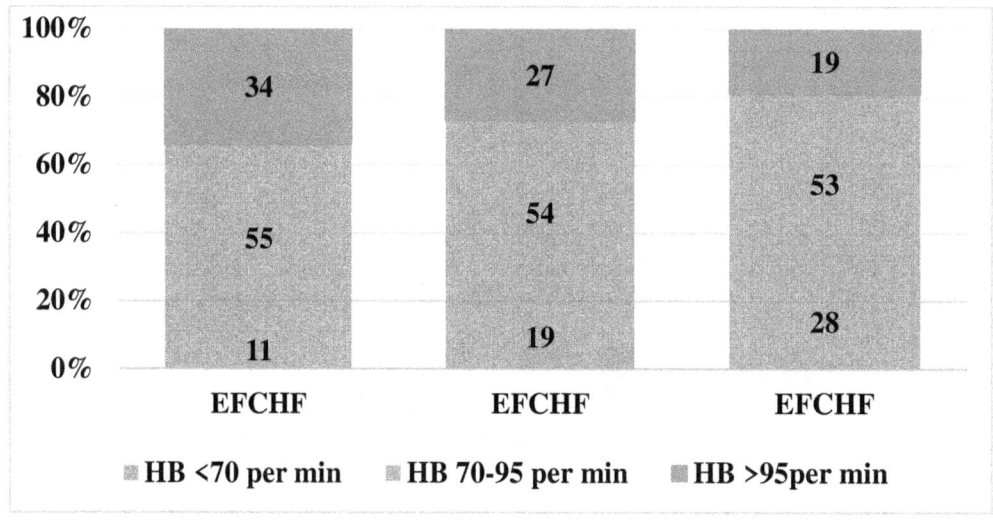

Note: Statistically significant difference when p < 0.05

**8 pictures. The number of initial heart contractions of patients depending on the phenotypes of the left ventricular ejection fraction.**

According to the results of the correlation analysis, there is a positive correlation between the patients' initial systolic arterial blood pressure and the left ventricular ejection fraction (r=0.186; P<0.05) and age (r=-0.172; P<0.05), between the amount of creatinine in the blood (r =-0.161; P<0.05) an inverse relationship was found. Diastolic arterial blood pressure is related to patients' age (r=0.194; P<0.05), body mass index (r=0.159; P<0.05), number of heart contractions (r=0.161; P<0.05), blood It was observed that the amount of creatinine (r=0.176; P<0.05) has a positive relationship with the glomerular filtration rate (r=0.170; P<0.05).

Thus, in patients with chronic heart failure with a preserved ejection fraction, high systolic and diastolic arterial blood pressure, a lower number of heart contractions are more characteristic in comparison to the cohort of patients with a reduced ejection fraction and a slightly reduced CHFli. In contrast, in patients with CHF, with a decrease in left ventricular ejection fraction, SABP, DABP tend to decrease, and HB tends to increase.

### 2.1.4. Results of laboratory tests

The amount of NT-proBNP increased with a decrease in left ventricular ejection fraction, and in patients with chronic heart failure with reduced ejection fraction, it was on average 3883±1214 pg/ml. There was no significant difference in creatine kinase MV, creatine kinase and troponin levels in CHF phenotypes according to left ventricular ejection fraction (Table 10).

**10 tables.**

**Quantification of NT-proBNP, creatine kinase, and troponin levels in CHF phenotypes.**

| Indicators | EFCHFn=54 | AEFCHF n=30 | OFCCHF n=36 |
|---|---|---|---|
| NT-proBNP | 3883±1214 | 3718±1146* | 3535±1016** |
| Creatine kinase, Ed/l | 134.5±36.0 | 105.2±29.0* | 124.8±37.0 |
| MV KFK, ED/l | 19.1±10.5 | 12.4±9.0* | 24.5±11.0 |
| Troponin, pg/ml | 0.04±0.007 | 0.03±0.004 | 0.05±0.002 |

Note: *r<0.05, r**<0.01 – patients with decreased firing fraction compared to the phenotype;

A positive correlation was found between the amount of NT-proBNP and the amount of creatinine (r=0.182; P<0.05) and potassium (r=0.162; P<0.05) and body mass index (r=-0.167; P<0, 05), triglycerides (r=-0.204; P<0.05), low-density lipoprotein cholesterol (r=-0.192; P<0.05), high-density lipoprotein cholesterol (r=-0.272; P<0.05), firing fraction, glomerular filtration rate (r=-0.572; P<0.05) were found to have an inverse relationship. NT-proBNP levels in patients with CHF with preserved firing fraction were found to be positively correlated with blood glucose levels (r=0.182; P<0.05). At the same time, no significant difference was observed between the lipid parameters and the phenotypes according to the CHF shoot fraction

When evaluating indicators of kidney function, it was observed that urea and creatinine levels were slightly higher in patients with EFCHF than in patients with AEFCHF and OFCCHF. At the same time, when assessing the rate of filtration of tubules, EFCHF, this indicator was observed to be relatively low (Table 11).

11 tables

**Indicators of kidney and liver function**

| Indicators | EFCHF n=54 | AEFCHF n=30 | OFCCHF n=36 |
|---|---|---|---|
| Urea, mmol/l | 9.1±4.2 | 8.2±3.9 | 7.7±3.6* |
| Creatinine, μmol/l | 124.0±22.8 | 115.0±19.7* | 107.4±16.8** |
| Ball filtration rate, ml/min, 1.73 m2 | 46.0±11.5 | 49.2±12.0 | 54.6±14.3** |
| ALT, ED/l | 27.4±8.2 | 25.1±7.4 | 21.6±6.1* |
| AST, ED/l | 33.8±14.0 | 29.4±12.2* | 24.1±11.0* |
| Bilirubin, μmol/l | 22.5±10.4 | 18.4±8.9* | 16.4±7.6* |

Note: *r<0.05, **r<0.01 – phenotype of patients with reduced firing fraction compared to

Elevated levels of liver enzymes were observed in patients with EFCHF. Alternatively, the phenotype of patients with CHF with preserved firing fraction was observed to have a low hemoglobin and erythrocyte count. Conversely, platelets and C-reactive protein levels tended to be higher in CHF patients with reduced firing fraction (Table 12).

12 tables

**Initial hematological indicators of patients.**

| Indicators | EFCHF n=54 | AEFCHF n=30 | OFCCHF |
|---|---|---|---|

|  |  |  | n=36 |
|---|---|---|---|
| Hemoglobin, g/ml | 141.0±24.2 | 135.2±21.7* | 128.0±19.4** |
| Erythrocyte, 10*12/l | 4.9±2.0 | 4.6±1.7 | 3.9±1.5* |
| Platelet, 10*9/l | 215.0±42.5 | 211.4±48.6 | 245.0±51.0 |
| Hematocrit, % | 42.0±8.1 | 37.4±7.1 | 33.5±5.4* |
| Leukocyte, 10*9/l | 5.8±2.4 | 5.9±1.9 | 5.7±2.2 |
| CRP, g/l | 37.3±10.5*** | 27.0±8.2** | 15.2±5.4 |

Note: *r<0.05, **r<0.01, ***r<0.001 – reduced firing fraction compared to the patients phenotype

Thus, with a decrease in the contractile activity of the myocardial CHF, there is an increase in the amount of heart failure biomarkers, kidney and liver enzymes.

### 2.1.5. Prehospital treatment of chronic heart failure

Before hospital visit, 62% of patients were taking beta blockers, 48% of patients were taking angiotensin-converting enzyme inhibitors, and 19% of patients were taking angiotensin receptor blockers. Furosemide 32%, torasemide 14%, mineralocorticoid receptor antagonists 31% took diuretic drugs. 6% of patients received thiazide diuretics. 16% of patients received cardiac glycosides and 28% of patients received statins. 21% of patients required nitrates. Patients with low ejection fraction were more likely to receive beta-blockers, renin-angiotensin-aldosterone system blockers, loop diuretics, and mineralocorticoid receptor antagonists. A quarter of these patients required cardiac glycosides. In patients with moderate ejection fraction, renin-angiotensin system blocker intake was similar to patients with preserved ejection fraction. At the same time, beta blockers and mineralocorticoid antagonists were almost the same as patients with preserved ejection fraction, while digoxin and diuretics were taken more by patients with chronic heart failure with a slightly reduced ejection fraction. Patients with AEFCHF received calcium antagonists in 7% of cases without taking thiazide diuretics (Table 13). In addition, most of the patients received antiaggregant drugs (79), antiarrhythmic and anticoagulant drugs in patients with heart rhythm disorders.

**13 tables**

**Admission of patients in the pre-hospital period the list of medications.**

| Indicators | CHF n=120 | EFCHF n=54 | AEFCHF n=30 | OFCCHF n=36 |
|---|---|---|---|---|
| ACEI (%) | 48 | 46 | 23* | 70** |
| ARB (%) | 19 | 15 | 17 | 30* |
| BB (%) | 62 | 57 | 33** | 69* |
| MRA (%) | 31 | 52 | 17** | 8*** |
| Digoxin (%) | 16 | 25 | 13* | 14* |
| Loop diuretics (%) | 46 | 52 | 43* | 39* |
| Thiazide diuretics (%) | 6 | 9 | - | 5 |
| Calcium antagonist (%) | 5 | 7 | 7 | 14* |
| Statins (%) | 28 | 24 | 30 | 36* |
| Nitrates (%) | 21 | 29 | 26 | 28 |
| Anticoagulant (%) | 41 | 18 | 11 | 12 |
| Antiarrhythmic (%) | 15 | 2 | 4 | 9* |
| Antiaggregant (%) | 79 | 36 | 19 | 24 |

Note:*r<0.05,**r<0.01,***r<0.001 phenotype of patients with reduced firing fraction compared to

In addition to beta blockers, diuretics and statins took the main place in the group of patients with preserved ejection fraction. Calcium antagonists and digoxin were included in the list of drugs taken in the least amount. Nitrates were almost uniformly accepted by patients with CHF of all phenotypes. The demand for angiotensin receptor blockers increased with the increase in firing fraction.

Thus, the drugs taken by patients with chronic heart failure in the pre-hospital period depend on the ejection fraction and concomitant diseases and do not fully comply with the standards.

## 2.1.6. Assessment of central hemodynamic indicators, myocardial condition and reserve of coronary arteries

Before randomization, ExoKG was performed to assess central hemodynamic parameters in all patients (Table 14). After that, the patients were divided into 3 phenotypic groups according to the indicator of firing fraction (Table 14). In patients with chronic heart failure with reduced ejection fraction, it was observed that the size of the left ventricle was larger than in patients with AEFCHF and OFCCHF (R<0.005). At the same time, significantly higher left ventricular end-diastolic size (ChQ SDO') and left ventricular end-systolic size (ChQ SSO') were observed in patients with this phenotype (R<0.005). It was found that the indicator of the linear integral velocity of the left ventricular outlet was significantly lower in patients with EFCHF (Table 15).

**14 tables**

**Patients' baseline echocardiographic parameters before randomization (M+SD)**

| Indicators | CHF n=120 |
|---|---|
| ChB, mm | 40.1±5.2 |
| ChQ SDO', mm | 67.4±18.6 |
| ChQ SSO', mm | 54.7±14.5 |
| ChQ firing fraction, % | 45.3±12.0 |
| Linear integral speed of the ChQ outlet, cm | 12.6±4.1 |
| ChQ SDH, ml/m2 | 132.4±42.8 |
| Assessment of tricuspid valve systolic excursion (TAPSE), mm | 19.4±4.9 |
| Maximum speed in the tricuspid loop, m/s | 3.2±1.1 |
| Pulmonary artery systolic pressure, mm.sm.ust. | 18.4±6.7 |
| yes | 18.1±7.5 |
| E/A | 1.7±0.4 |
| Interventricular barrier size, mm | 1.24±0.34 |
| The size of the thickness of the left ventricle, mm | 1.21±0.36 |
| Left ventricular weight index, g/m2 | 119.4±31.5 |
| Summary index of left ventricular contractility | 2.95±0.48 |

| Summary index of left ventricular contractility after stress echocardiography with dobutamine | 2.3±0.68 |
|---|---|

Note: ChB – left part; ChQ SDO' – left ventricular end-diastolic size; ChQ SSO' – left ventricular end-diastolic size; ChQ SDH – left ventricular end-diastolic volume;

**15 tables**

## Baseline echocardiographic parameters of patients according to left ventricular ejection fraction phenotypes

| Indicators | EFCHF n=54 | AEFCHF n=30 | OFCCHF n=36 |
|---|---|---|---|
| ChB, mm | 42.2±4.7 | 40.0±5.6 | 38.2±5.8* |
| ChQ SDO', mm | 85.4±19.6 | 76.0±19.0* | 64.1±18.0* |
| ChQ SSO', mm | 61.2±15.5 | 55.7±14.4* | 53.7±14.7* |
| ChQ firing fraction, % | 38.2±12.0 | 45.2±11.9 | 52.5±12.6* |
| Linear integral speed of the ChQ outlet, cm | 10.2±3.9 | 14.2±6.7** | 15.6±8.1** |
| ChQ SDH, ml/m2 | 148±42.8 | 122.4±42.8* | 115.3±37.9* |
| Assessment of tricuspid valve systolic excursion (TAPSE), mm | 13.4±4.1 | 16.1±4.5 | 21.0±5.2* |
| Three-layer maximum speed, m/s | 3.5±1.3 | 3.3±1.2 | 3.0±1.0* |
| Pulmonary artery systolic pressure, mm.sm.ust. | 21.8±6.7 | 17.2±6.3 | 14.3±6.1* |
| yes | 19.1±7.5 | 16.1±6.6 | 14.2±5.9* |
| E/A | 1.9±0.5 | 1.8±0.6 | 1.6±0.3 |
| Interventricular barrier size, mm | 1.21±0.34 | 1.28±0.38 | 1.20±0.28 |
| The size of the thickness of the back wall of the left ventricle, mm | 1.17±0.36 | 1.21±0.38 | 1.28±0.39 |
| Left ventricular weight index, g/m2 | 124.4±32.2 | 118.2±32.6 | 116.4±30.1* |
| Summary index of left ventricular contractility | 2.79±0.45 | 3.04±0.54 | 3.12±0.64* |
| Summary index of left ventricular | 2.1±0.57 | 2.6±0.75 | 2.8±0.94* |

| contractility after stress echocardiography with dobutamine | | . | |

Note: *p<0.05, **p<0.01– phenotype of patients with reduced firing fraction compared to

Left ventricular end-systolic and diastolic volumes increased with decreasing ejection fraction and were observed to be the highest in patients with EFCHF. Tricuspid valve systolic excursion was observed to be the highest in patients with OFCCHF compared to other phenotypes (R<0.05). Pulmonary artery systolic pressure increased with a decrease in ejection fraction. Although E/e' increased with decreasing firing fraction, no difference was observed between E/A values. There was no significant difference (R>0.05) between the size of the interventricular barrier and left ventricular thickness depending on the ejection fraction phenotypes. The left ventricular weight index was lower in patients with CHF with preserved ejection fraction, but the sum index of left ventricular contractility was higher. The summary index of left ventricular contractility after stress echocardiography with dobutamine was also observed to be higher in patients with chronic heart failure with preserved ejection fraction. As can be seen from the above, the central hemodynamic parameters change according to a certain regularity depending on the ejection fraction of the left ventricle.

When the reserve of coronary arteries was studied separately for the phenotypes of changes in left ventricular ejection fraction, it was observed that the reserve volume of coronary arteries in patients with OFCCHF was slightly higher in the anterior descending coronary artery and in the right coronary artery than in patients with EFCHF and patients with OFbsCHF. In addition, no differences were observed between firing fraction phenotypes when the relative reserve volume of coronary arteries was evaluated (Table 16).

**16 tables**

**Assessment of coronary artery reserve**

| Indicators | CHF n=120 | EFCHF n=54 | AEFCHF n=30 | OFCCHF n=36 |
|---|---|---|---|---|

| | | | | |
|---|---|---|---|---|
| VpdPNA (stress)mm.sm.ust. | 89±24 | 84±22 | 91±24 | 97±26* |
| VpdPNA (at rest) mm.sm.ust. | 60.5±25 | 60±20 | 61±24 | 61±28 |
| TAZ PNA | 1.5±0.4 | 1.4±0.4 | 1.5±0.5 | 1.6±0.7* |
| VpdPKA (stress) mm.sm.ust. | 82±19 | 83±17 | 86±20 | 93±21* |
| VpdPKA (at rest) mm.sm.ust. | 66±16 | 70±19 | 73±21 | 75±19 |
| TAZ PKA | 1.25±0.4 | 1.15±0.4 | 1.19±0.64* | 1.24±0.82** |
| Relative reserve volume of coronary arteries | 1.15±0.4 | 1.2±0.4 | 1.1±0.35 | 1.1±0.42 |

Note: *$p<0.05$, **$p<0.01$ – when compared with the phenotype of patients with reduced firing fraction; Vpd is the highest blood flow rate (pressure) in diastole; PNA - anterior descending artery; TAZ - reserve volume of coronary artery; PKA - right coronary artery.

As can be seen from the table above, coronary artery reserve volume is higher in the contingent of patients with preserved ejection fraction and has a relatively stable reserve in the dipyridamole stress test.

### 2.2. Assessment of the activity of the sodium-uretic peptide system and the structural and functional state of the myocardium in patients with CHF

When BNP and NT-proBNP were analyzed as biomarkers of chronic heart failure, it was observed that these biomarkers are related to central hemodynamic indicators, ie echocardiographic indicators of the heart. It was found that the left ventricular ejection fraction indicator is inversely related to BNP and NT-proBNP, chronic heart failure biomarkers were found to increase with a decrease in the left ventricular ejection fraction, and according to the results of the analysis, these biomarkers were inversely related to the left ventricular ejection fraction ($r=-0.85$, CI 95%, $R<0.05$; 10, 11 pictures).

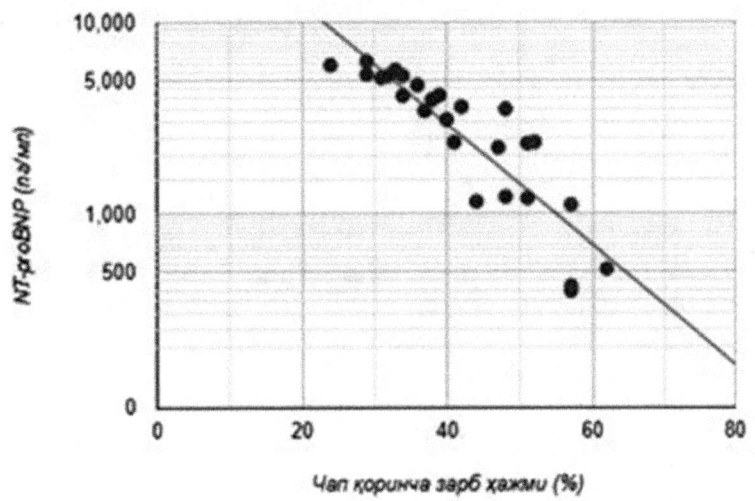

Note: Statistically significant difference when p < 0.05

**10 pictures. Association between NT-proBNP activity and left ventricular stroke volume in chronic heart failure**

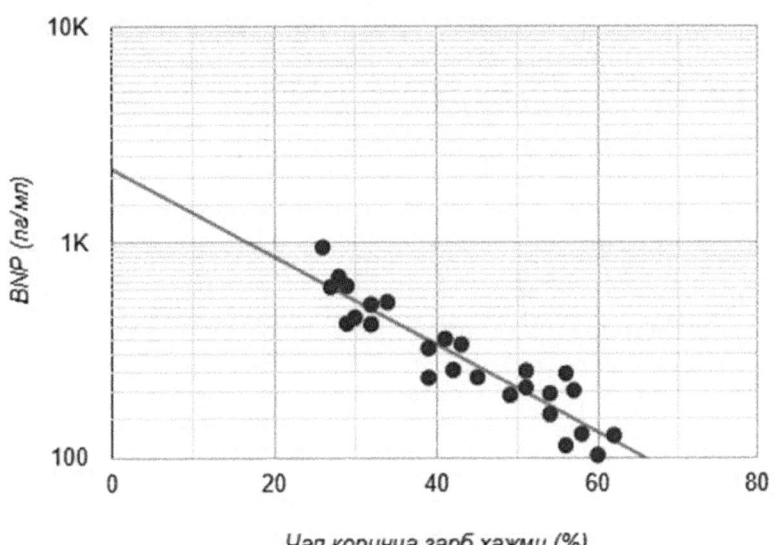

Note: Statistically significant difference when p < 0.05

**11 pictures. Relationship between BNP activity and left ventricular stroke volume in chronic heart failure**

When the relationship between BNP and NT-proBNP biomarkers of chronic heart failure and left ventricular size was analyzed, it was observed that the left ventricular size was correctly associated with the above biomarkers. In particular, the amount of BNP and NT-proBNP in plasma increased as the size of the left lobe increased (r=0.85; II 95%; R<0.05; for BNP and r=0.78; II 95%; R<0 ,05; for NT-proBNP; Figures 12, 13).

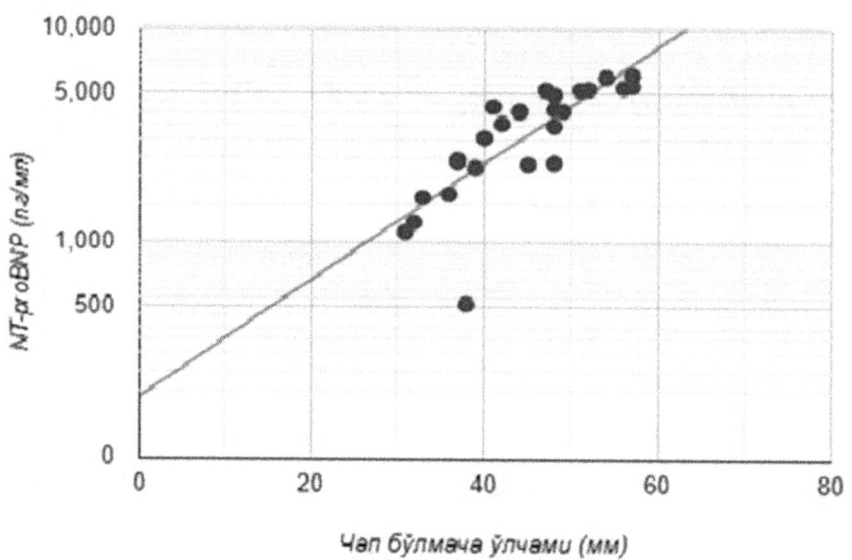

Note: Statistically significant difference when p < 0.05

**12 pictures. Association between NT-proBNP activity and left ventricular size in chronic heart failure**

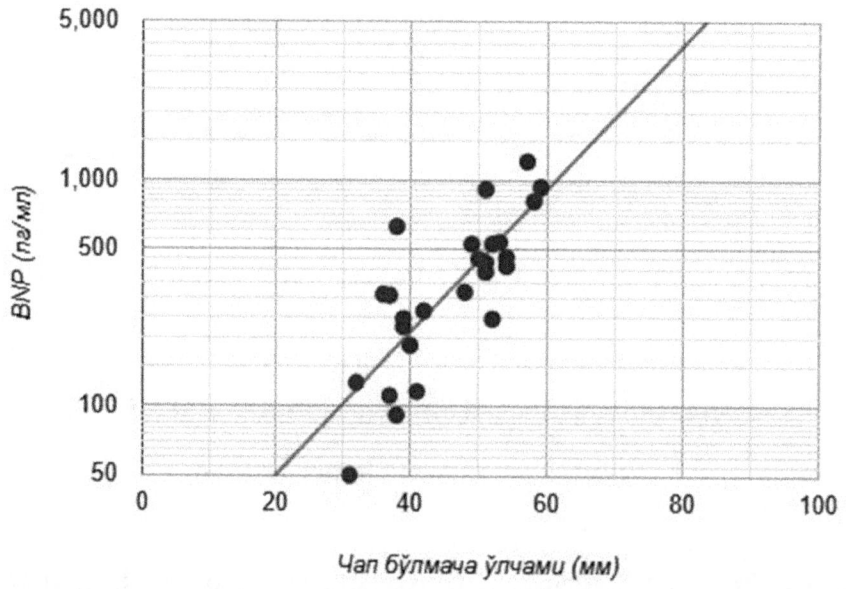

Note: Statistically significant difference when p < 0.05

**13 pictures. Association between BNP activity and left ventricular size in chronic heart failure**

When examining the relationship between left ventricular aftersystolic and diastolic size from central hemodynamic parameters and biomarkers of chronic heart failure, an increase in NT-proBNP was observed in parallel with an increase in left ventricular aftersystolic and diastolic size (r=0.71; II 95%; 14 , 15 pictures).

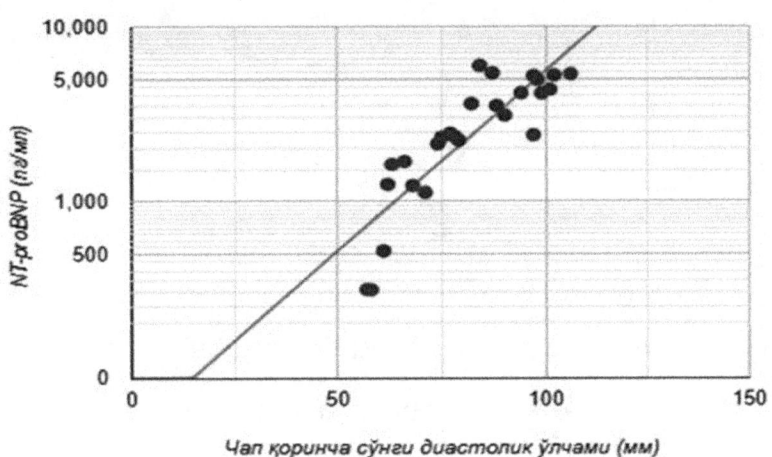

Note: Statistically significant difference when p < 0.05

**14 pictures. Association between NT-proBNP activity and left ventricular end-diastolic size in chronic heart failure**

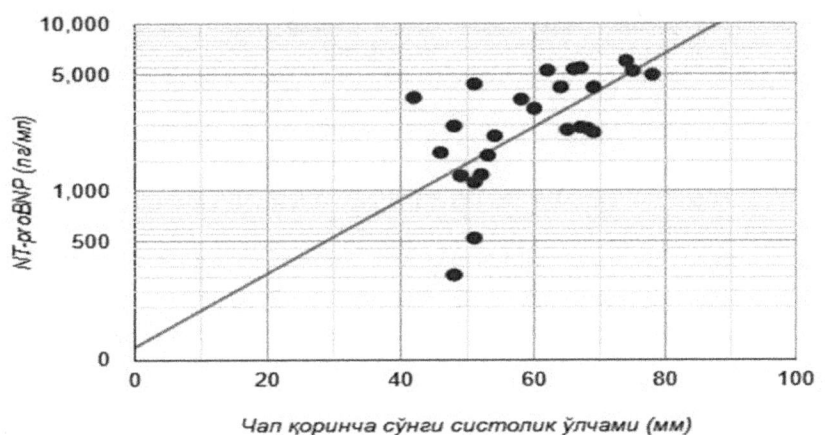

Note: Statistically significant difference when p < 0.05

**15 pictures. Association between NT-proBNP activity and left ventricular end-systolic size in chronic heart failure**

When the relationship between left ventricular end-systolic and diastolic size and BNP was studied, it was found that there is a correct relationship between them, that is, as the left ventricular end-systolic and diastolic size increases, the concentration of BNP in plasma increases (r=0.68; II 95%; 16, 17 pictures).

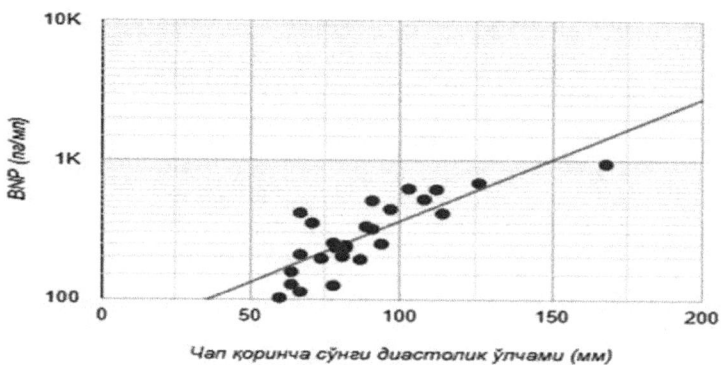

Note: Statistically significant difference when p < 0.05

**16 pictures. Association between BNP activity and left ventricular end-diastolic size in chronic heart failure**

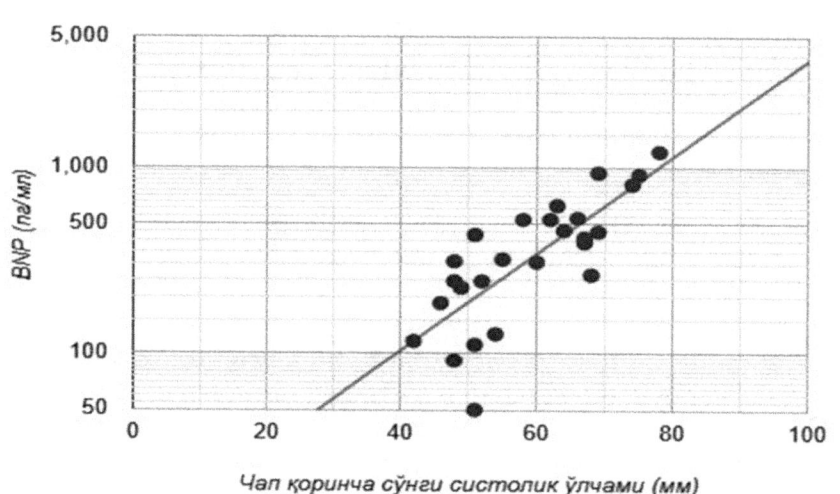

Note: Statistically significant difference when p < 0.05

**17 pictures. Association between BNP activity and left ventricular end-systolic size in chronic heart failure**

When the relationship between the linear integral velocity of the left ventricular output and biomarkers of chronic heart failure was studied, no significant relationship was observed between them. When left ventricular end-diastolic volume and CHF biomarkers were studied, a weak positive association was found between them. With the increase in the end-diastolic volume of the left ventricle, the concentration of BNP in the plasma tended to increase (r=0.52; II 95%; Fig. 16). In addition, with the increase in the end-diastolic volume of the left ventricle, the amount of NT-proBNP in the plasma also increased (r=0.57; II 95%; pictures 18, 19).

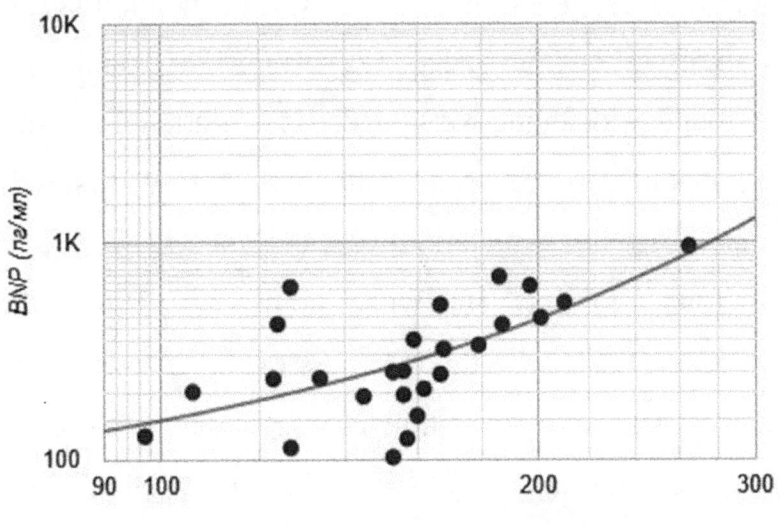

Note: Statistically significant difference when p < 0.05

**Figure 18. Relationship between BNP activity and left ventricular end-diastolic volume in chronic heart failure**

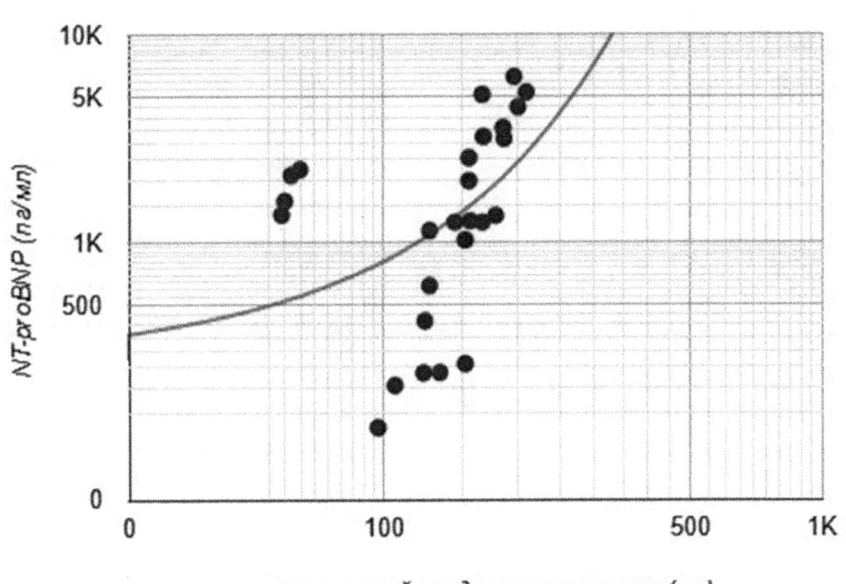

Note: Statistically significant difference when p < 0.05

**19 pictures. Association between NT-proBNP activity and left ventricular end-diastolic volume in chronic heart failure**

When tricuspid valve blood flow parameters, including tricuspid valve systolic excursion and tricuspid annulus peak velocity, were examined, no significant association was found with biomarkers of chronic heart failure. In addition, when examining the relationship between pulmonary artery systolic pressure and biomarkers, no clear signs of association were observed between them. Neither E/e' nor E/A were found to correlate with biomarkers. When the size of the interventricular barrier, the size of the thickness of the left ventricle and the weight index of the left ventricle were studied, there was no significant correlation of these parameters with the biomarkers (P>0.05). When studying the correlation of biomarkers with the summary index of left ventricular contractility, it was found that there is an inverse relationship between them (r=-0.62; II 95%; Figures 20, 21).

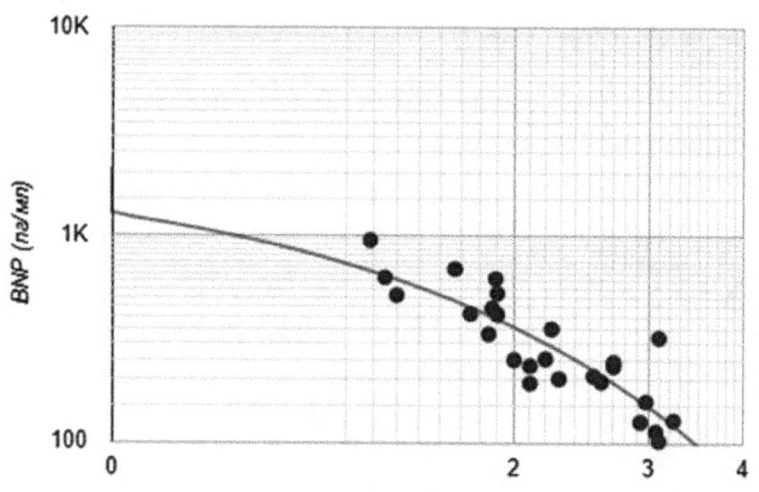

Note: Statistically significant difference when p < 0.05

**20 pictures. Association between BNP activity and the summary index of left ventricular contractility in chronic heart failure**

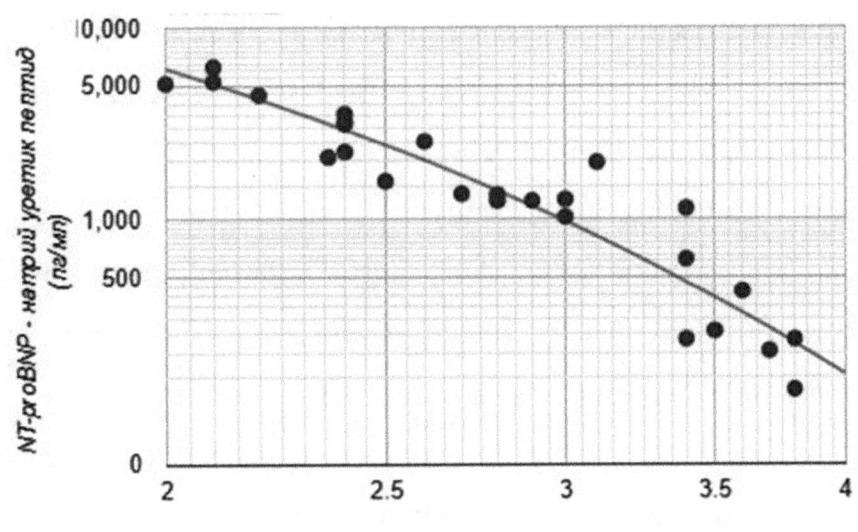

Note: Statistically significant difference when p < 0.05

**21 pictures. Association between NT-proBNP (Natriuretic Peptide) Activity and Summary Index of Left Ventricular Contractility in Chronic Heart Failure**

In conclusion, plasma concentrations of BNP and NT-proBNP as biomarkers of chronic heart failure have a positive relationship with left ventricular size, left ventricular systolic and diastolic dimensions, and left ventricular end-diastolic volume. Left ventricular ejection fraction, and the sum index of left ventricular contractility were found to have an inverse relationship between plasma concentrations of BNP and NT-proBNP.

# EVALUATION OF THE EFFICACY OF A 12-WEEK SACUBITRIL/VALSARTAN TREATMENT IN PATIENTS WITH CHF

- 3.1. Clinical demographics of patients.

The patients involved in the study were divided into 2 groups by simple randomization, i.e. 1 group received sacubitril/valsartan on the background of standard treatment (a small dose of 26/24 mg was prescribed 2 times, the dose was titrated up to the maximum tolerated dose of 103/97 mg), the next group received only valsartan on the background of standard treatment took the drug (starting at a low dose of 40mg and titrated up to a maximum tolerated dose of 160mg). Of these, 25 patients remained on sacubitril/valsartan 24/26 mg, 22 patients increased to 51/49 mg, and 13 patients increased to 103/97 mg based on baseline blood pressure readings and drug tolerance. Of the patients in the valsartan group, 21 remained on valsartan 40 mg, 19 on valsartan 80 mg, and 20 on valsartan 160 mg. Both groups were observed to have similar baseline patient demographics. Table 11 shows the initial clinical demographics of the patients in the groups. The average age of patients in group 1 was 67.6±11.9 years, and the average age in group 2 was 68.3±12.4 years. In the sacubitril/valsartan group, 48% of patients were women and 52% were men, while in the 2 groups, women and men were 50%. The body weight index of patients in the first group was 30.2±8.0 kg/m2, and in the second group it was 31.4±7.8 kg/m2. 20% of patients in the sacubitril/valsartan group were smokers, and 17% of patients in the valsartan group were smokers. Alcohol consumption was similar in both groups, including 8 patients in group 1 consumed alcohol, while 7 patients in group 2 consumed alcohol. 77% of patients in group 1 had a history of myocardial infarction, and 63% of patients in group 2 had it. Percutaneous coronary intervention was performed in 6 patients in the sacubitril/valsartan group and in 8 patients in the valsartan group. Aortic coronary bypass surgery was observed in 13% of patients in group 1, and in 8% of patients in group 2. Associated arterial hypertension was observed in 91% of patients in group 1, and in 90% of patients in group 2. In the sacubitril/valsartan group, compartmental tremor was observed in 21 patients due to comorbidities, complications after BMQAO'B in 17% of patients, SBK in 25% of patients, and anemia in 25% of patients. Charlson scale averaged 7.2±2.4 in group 1, and 7.0±3.4 in group 2 (Table 17).

17 tables

**Clinical demographic characteristics of patients with chronic heart failure according to treatment groups**

| Indicator | 1 group Sacubitril/valsartan n=60 | 2 groups Valsartan n=60 | R value |
|---|---|---|---|
| Age, year | 67.6±11.9 | 68.3±12.4 | >0.05 |
| Gender male/female, (%) | (48)/(52) | (50)/(50) | >0.05 |
| TMI, kg/m2 | 30.2±8.0 | 31.4±7.8 | >0.05 |
| Smoking, n(%) | 12 (20) | 10 (17) | >0.05 |
| Alcohol, n(%) | 8 (13) | 7 (11) | >0.05 |
| Angina: FC II | 16 (13.3) | 20 (16.7) | >0.05 |
| FC III | 23 (19.2) | 21 (17.5) | >0.05 |
| FC IV | 21 (17.5) | 19 (15.8) | >0.05 |
| IKKS, n(%) | 46 (77) | 38 (63) | >0.05 |
| Percutaneous coronary intervention, n(%) | 6 (10) | 8 (13) | >0.05 |
| In US anamnesis, n(%) | 8 (13) | 4 (8) | >0.05 |
| Arterial hypertension, n(%) | 55 (91) | 54 (90) | >0.05 |
| Diabetes, n(%) | 26 (43) | 23 (40) | >0.05 |
| Volatility constant form of fractions, n(%) | 21 (35) | 20 (33) | >0.05 |
| Status after UNFCCC, n(%) | 10 (17) | 11 (18) | >0.05 |
| SBK, n(%) | 15 (25) | 17 (28) | >0.05 |
| Anemia, n(%) | 15 (25) | 13 (22) | >0.05 |
| OSOK, n(%) | 11 (18) | 15 (25) | >0.05 |

| Charlson scale | 7.2±2.4 | 7.0±3.4 | >0.05 |
|---|---|---|---|

• 3.2. In the groups, patients' initial clinical and **hemodynamic indicators.**

In the examination, 78% of patients in group 1 had symptoms such as panting during physical activity, swelling in legs in 80%, fatigue in 48%, and weakness in 83% of patients in group 2, panting at rest in 45%, panting during physical exertion in 85%, and swelling in 78%. . Half of the patients in the first group had signs of hemostasis according to X-ray examination, while in the second group this indicator was 48%. However, there was no significant difference in clinical signs between the two groups (Table 18).

**18 tables**

**Patients with chronic heart failure clinical symptoms (n=120)**

| Indicator | 1 group n=60 | 2 groups n=60 | R value is n=30 |
|---|---|---|---|
| Fatigue, n (%) | 47 (78%) | 50 (83%) | >0.05 |
| Wheezing at rest, n (%) | 29 (48%) | 27 (45%) | >0.05 |
| Panting during physical exertion, n (%) | 56 (93%) | 51 (85%) | >0.05 |
| Orthopnea, n (%) | 23 (38%) | 21 (35%) | >0.05 |
| Tumors, n (%) | 48 (80%) | 47 (78%) | >0.05 |
| Wheezing in the lungs, n (%) | 36 (60%) | 35 (58%) | >0.05 |
| Hepatomegaly, n (%) | 26 (43%) | 24 (40%) | >0.05 |
| Signs of hemostasis according to X-ray examination, n (%) | 30 (50%) | 29 (48%) | >0.05 |

Among patients in the sacubitril/valsartan group, chronic heart failure was 30% of patients with NYHA II FC, compared with 28% in the valsartan group. According to NYHA, 40% of patients with FC III in group 1 and 43% in group 2 were observed. According to NYHA, patients with IV FC were found to be 30% in group 1 and 28%

in group 2. But when the groups were compared, there was no significant difference between the NYHA functional classes of chronic heart failure between the groups (Figure 22).

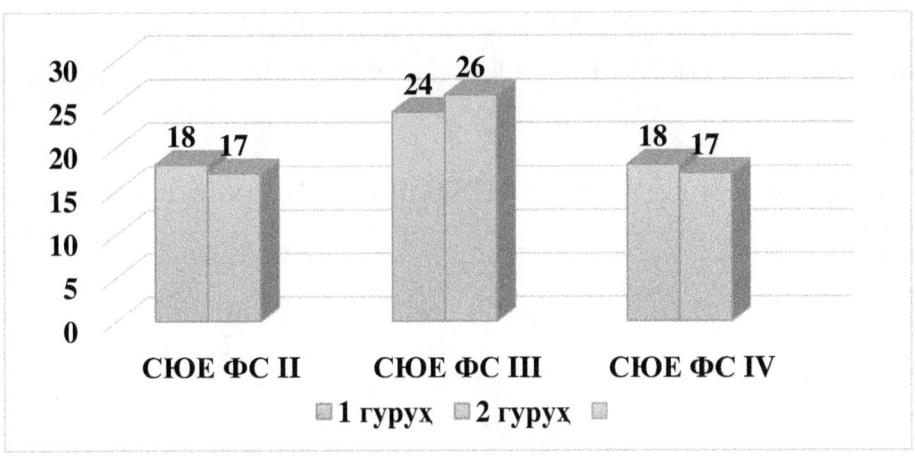

Note: Statistically significant difference when p < 0.05

**22 pictures. Distribution of NYHA functional classes of primary chronic heart failure among patients between groups.**

According to the results of a 6-minute test conducted on patients, the average distance covered in the first examination in patients with chronic heart failure in group 1 was 206.4±38.0 meters, and in patients in group 2 it was 212.5±66.3 meters. In addition, the index of minute oxygen consumption in the first examination was 12.8±6.2 ml/(kgxmin) in group 1, and 13.1±6.4 ml/(kgxmin) in group 2 (Figure 23).

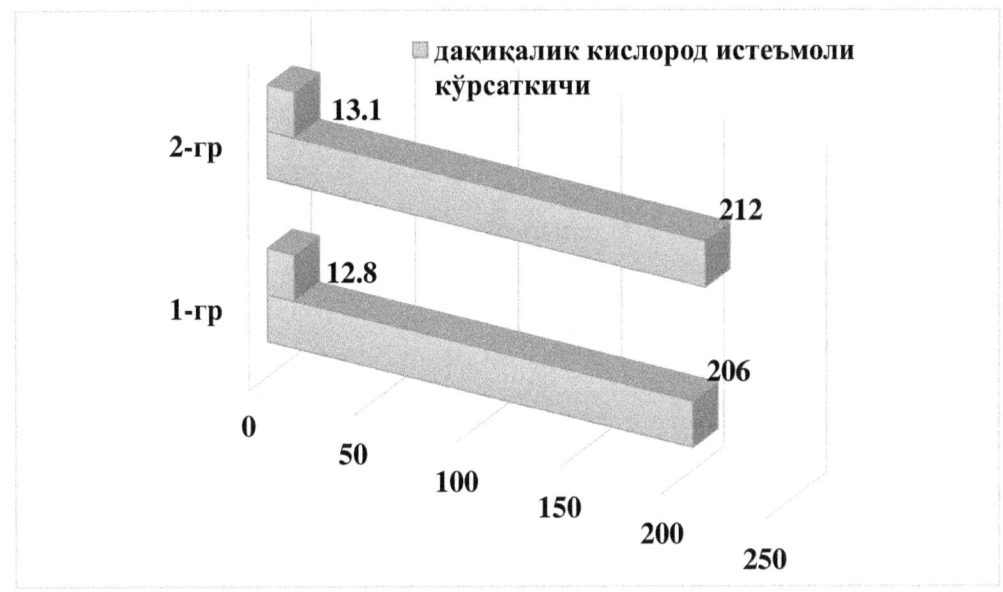

Note: Statistically significant difference when p < 0.05

**23 pictures. Distance traveled during the first 6-minute trial and minute oxygen demand between groups.**

When hemodynamic indicators of patients were analyzed, arterial blood pressure and the number of heart contractions were similar in both groups (Table 19).

**19 tables**

**SAKB and DAKB as well as UKB and YuKS pointers in groups**

| Indicators | 1 group n=60 | 2 groups n=60 | R value |
|---|---|---|---|
| SABP, mm.sm.ust. | 129.6±19.2 | 131.6±24.5 | >0.05 |
| DABP, , mm.sm.ust. | 78.9±12.4 | 79.0±14.1 | >0.05 |
| Average ABP, mm.cm.asl. | 108.8±14.4 | 109.1±16.2 | >0.05 |
| HIGH, th/min | 85.4±22.0 | 86.6±25.8 | >0.05 |

- 3.3. Preliminary laboratory of patients in groups

**inspection indicators.**

At baseline, NT-proBNP was 3812±1326 pg/ml in the sacubitril/valsartan group and 3612±1287 pg/ml in the valsartan group, but there was no significant difference between the two groups (R>0.05). In addition, the mean concentration of BNP in plasma was 512±46 pg/ml in group 1 and 498±52 pg/ml in group 2, and the change in both groups was not statistically significant (Table 20).

**20 tables**

**NT-proBNP, amount of BNP in groups**

| Indicators | 1 group=60 | 2 groups n=60 | R value |
|---|---|---|---|
| NT-proBNP | 3812±1326 | 3612±1287 | >0.05 |
| BNP | 512±46 | 498±52 | >0.05 |

Table 21 shows the range of baseline lipid values between groups. As can be seen from the table, there was no significant difference between the groups in terms of initial indicators.

**21 tables**

**Quantification of lipid parameters between the initial groups**

| Indicators | 1 group n=60 | 2 groups n=60 | R value |
|---|---|---|---|
| Total cholesterol, mmol/l | 5.1±1.7 | 4.9±1.9 | >0.05 |
| Triglyceride, mmol/l | 3.5±1.6 | 3.7±2.0 | >0.05 |
| Low-density lipoprotein cholesterol, mmol/l | 3.1±1.9 | 3.2±2.0 | >0.05 |
| High-density lipoprotein cholesterol, mmol/l | 1.2±0.6 | 1.1±0.8 | >0.05 |

When the indicators of kidney function were evaluated, the urea and creatinine levels of patients in group 1 tended to be slightly higher than those in group 2, but there was no statistically significant difference (>0.05). Preliminary comparative analysis between groups is detailed in Table 16 (Table 22).

**22 tables**

**Indicators of kidney and liver function.**

| Indicators | 1 group=60 | 2 groups n=60 | R value |
|---|---|---|---|
| Urea, mmol/l | 9.0±4.6 | 8.9±4.8 | >0.05 |
| Creatinine, µmol/l | 121.0±24.4 | 118.0±21.9 | >0.05 |
| Ball filtration rate, ml/min, 1.73 m2 | 48.0±12.5 | 49.2±12.0 | >0.05 |
| ALT, ED/l | 22.4±9.2 | 25.1±7.4 | >0.05 |
| AST, ED/l | 24.8±14.0 | 26.4±12.2 | >0.05 |
| Bilirubin, µmol/l | 2215±10.4 | 18.4±8.9* | >0.05 |

Note: *r<0.05– when compared with the phenotype of patients with reduced firing fraction

When the parameters of the general blood analysis were evaluated, it was observed that the initial parameters were similar in the sacubitril/valsartan and valsartan groups (>0.05). Blood general analysis results It is detailed in Table 23.

**23 tables**

**Initial hematological indicators of patients**

| Indicators | 1 group=60 | 2 groups n=60 | R value |
|---|---|---|---|
| Hemoglobin, g/ml | 138.0±26.2 | 135.7±24.7 | >0.05 |
| Erythrocyte, 10*12/l | 4.3±2.0 | 4.1±1.8 | >0.05 |
| Platelet, 10*9/l | 212.0±42.5 | 210.4±48.9 | >0.05 |
| Hematocrit, % | 40.0±8.1 | 37.4±7.5 | >0.05 |
| Leukocyte, 10*9/l | 5.6±2.2 | 5.7±1.9 | >0.05 |
| CRP, g/l | 18.2±5.8 | 20.0±8.0 | >0.05 |

Thus, in the initial examination, the indicators were similar in both groups, and no significant differences were observed between them (>0.05).

### 3.3.1. Pre-hospital treatment of patients in groups.

Before visiting the hospital, 47% of patients in group 1 received ACEI inhibitors, while in group 2 this figure was 49%. Angiotensin receptor blockers were also taken in similar amounts in both groups. The most popular beta blocker was observed in 65% of patients in group 1, and in 59% of patients in group 2. Among other drugs, no significant difference was observed between the two groups (P>0.05, Table 24 shows the pre-hospital drugs of the patients between the groups. .

**24 tables**

**List of drugs taken by patients in groups before hospitalization**

| Indicators | 1 group=60 | 2 groups=60 | R value |
|---|---|---|---|
| ACEI (%) | 47 | 49 | >0.05 |
| ARB (%) | 18 | 17 | >0.05 |
| BB (%) | 65 | 59* | <0.05 |
| MRA (%) | 41 | 38 | >0.05 |
| Digoxin (%) | 19 | 21 | >0.05 |
| Loop diuretics (%) | 42 | 49* | >0.05 |
| Thiazide diuretics (%) | 5 | 7 | >0.05 |
| Calcium antagonist (%) | 3 | 4 | >0.05 |
| Statins (%) | 25 | 27 | >0.05 |
| Nitrates (%) | 23 | 25 | >0.05 |
| Anticoagulants (%) | 33 | 35 | >0.05 |

| Antiaggregants (%) | 77 | 81 | >0.05 |
| Antiarrhythmics (%) | 17 | 13 | >0.05 |

Note: *r<0.05– when compared with the phenotype of patients with reduced firing fraction

### 3.3.2. Indicators of initial coronary reserve and myocardial condition of patients in groups

In the sacubitril/valsartan group, the left ventricular size at baseline was 43.0±4.5 cm, compared with 42.5±4.9 cm in the valsartan group (R>0.05). The end-diastolic size of the left ventricle in group 1 was 66.3±17.4mm at the initial examination, and it was observed that it was less than that of the second group, but the differences were not statistically significant. In addition, left ventricular end-systolic size, left ventricular end-diastolic volume, maximum velocity in the tricuspid annulus, systolic blood pressure in the pulmonary artery, E/e', E/A and the summary index of left ventricular contractility after stress echocardiography with dobutamine were slightly lower compared to the valsartan group. but no statistically significant differences were observed (25- table). In addition, in the initial examination, the linear integral velocity of the left ventricular outflow tract, TAPSE index, interventricular barrier size, left ventricular thickness, left ventricular weight index, left ventricular contractility summary index tended to be slightly higher in the first group of patients, but no statistically significant difference was detected between them. (P>0.05).

**25 tables**

**Initial echocardiographic indicators of patients in groups**

| Indicators | 1 group n=60 | 2 groups n=60 | R value |
|---|---|---|---|
| ChB, cm | 43.0±4.5 | 42.5±4.9 | 0.198 |
| ChQ SDO', mm | 66.3±17.4 | 69.4±18.2 | 0.214 |
| ChQ SSO', mm | 54.2±14.5 | 58.4±15.5 | 0.080 |
| ChQ firing fraction, % | 42.2±12.0 | 43.1±11.9 | 0.048** |
| Linear integral speed of the ChQ outlet, cm | 14.0±4.6 | 12.1±4.4 | 0.245 |
| ChQ SDH, ml/m2 | 136.0±41.5 | 144.0±43.8 | 0.350 |
| Assessment of tricuspid valve | 18.1±4.7 | 15.4±4.3 | 0.070 |

| systolic excursion (TAPSE), mm | | | |
|---|---|---|---|
| Maximum speed in the tricuspid loop, m/s | 3.3±1.2 | 3.6±1.4 | 0.278 |
| Pulmonary artery systolic pressure, mm.sm.ust. | 18.1±6.7 | 19.8±6.9 | 0.249 |
| yes | 17.2±6.6 | 18.3±7.0 | 0.195 |
| E/A | 1.6±0.5 | 1.8±0.6 | 0.090 |
| Interventricular barrier size, mm | 1.29±0.36 | 1.25±0.35 | 0.210 |
| The size of the thickness of the left ventricle, mm | 1.28±0.38 | 1.19±0.33 | 0.315 |
| Left ventricular weight index, g/m2 | 124.4±32.5 | 122.4±35.0 | 0.165 |
| Summary index of left ventricular contractility | 2.98±0.49 | 2.79±0.46 | 0.085 |
| Summary index of left ventricular contractility after stress echocardiography with dobutamine | 2.2±0.69 | 2.3±0.68 | 0.148 |

Note: **r<0.05– compared with the phenotype of patients with reduced firing fraction

No significant changes were observed in both groups when the reserve volume of the coronary arteries was evaluated at the initial examination of the patients. In particular, peak diastolic blood flow velocity during stress diastole with dipyridamole test of anterior descending coronary artery was 88.0±23.0 mmHg in the sacubitril/valsartan group and 85.2±21.3 mmHg in the valsartan group at baseline. was equal to .sm.ust., but there was no statistically significant difference between the groups. At the same time, the highest blood flow velocity of the anterior descending coronary artery in rest diastole was 61.5±25, mm.cm.ust in the initial examination. was equal to and slightly higher than the valsartan group (59.4±20.3 mm Hg), but no statistical differences were observed between the groups (0.120). Coronary artery reserve volume was slightly higher in the sacubitril/valsartan group than in the 2 groups, but these differences were not statistically significant (0.064). In addition, stress and resting diastolic peak blood flow velocity and reserve volume of the right coronary artery were similar in the initial examination in both groups (P>0.05). In addition, the relative reserve volume of the coronary arteries was not significantly different between the groups at baseline (Table 26).

**26 tables**

**Assessment of coronary artery reserve**

| Indicators | 1 group=60 | 2 groups=60 | R value |
|---|---|---|---|
| VpdPNA (stress)mm.sm.ust. | 88.0±23.0 | 85.2±21.3 | 0.075 |
| VpdPNA (at rest) mm.sm.ust. | 61.5±25.0 | 59.4±20.3 | 0.120 |
| TAZ PNA | 1.6±0.4 | 1.4±0.35 | 0.064 |
| VpdPKA (stress) mm.sm.ust. | 83.2±19.4 | 82.8±17.9 | 0.069 |
| VpdPKA (at rest) mm.sm.ust. | 68.0±16.0 | 65.2±19.4 | 0.058 |
| TAZ PKA | 1.22±0.45 | 1.29±0.6 | 0.075 |
| Relative reserve volume of coronary arteries | 1.15±0.4 | 1.18±0.6 | 0.125 |

Note: statistically significant difference when p<0.05; Vpd is the highest blood flow rate (pressure) in diastole; PNA - anterior descending artery; TAZ - reserve volume of coronary artery; PKA - right coronary artery.

As can be seen from the table above, the total and relative reserve volumes of the coronary arteries were similar in both groups at baseline.

### • 3.4. Efficacy, safety, and effects on clinical and biochemical parameters of 12-week treatment with sacubitril/valsartan

The use of sacubitril/valsartan drug had a positive effect on the subjective condition of patients. This positive effect was especially evident in patients suffering from shortness of breath (Table 21). In particular, fatigue decreased from 78% to 17% in group 1 patients, and this indicator increased from 83% to 43% in the valsartan group (R<0.05), that is, in both groups, fatigue was significantly reduced on the background of treatment, but when we compared the groups, the differences in the first group it was observed that it was significant in patients (R<0.05). In addition, wheezing at rest showed significant changes in patients in both groups during treatment, including 48% of patients in the sacubitril/valsartan group had wheezing at rest at baseline, but only 8% of patients had wheezing at rest after 3 months of treatment (R<0.05). In the valsartan group, 45% of patients had wheezing at rest during the initial examination, while only 15% of patients suffered from this complaint during treatment (R<0.05). Although there was a significant reduction in complaints during treatment in both groups, these changes were observed to be significant in the sacubitril/valsartan group (R<0.05). In group 1, panting during exercise decreased from 93% to 27%, and in group 2, it decreased from 85% to 47% (R<0.05). In addition, other subjective clinical signs also showed significant changes in both groups on the background of treatment, but there was no statistically significant change between groups (R>0.05). Table 27 details the effect of sacubitril/valsartan and valsartan groups on subjective complaints of patients.

**27 tables**

**Changes of clinical signs in groups against the background of treatment**

| Indicator | 1 group (sacubitril/valsartan) n=60 | | 2 groups (valsartan) n=60 | | R value |
|---|---|---|---|---|---|
| | Initial indicator | Post-treatment performance | Initial indicator | Post-treatment performance | |
| Fatigue, n (%) | 47 (78%) | 17 (28%) | 50 (83%) | 26 (43%) | <0.05 |
| Wheezing at rest, n(%) | 29 (48%) | 5 (8%) | 27 (45%) | 9 (15%) | <0.05 |
| Panting during physical exertion, n (%) | 56 (93%) | 16 (27%) | 51 (85%) | 28 (47%) | <0.05 |
| Orthopnea, n (%) | 23 (38%) | 0 (0%) | 21 (35%) | 2 (3%) | >0.05 |
| Tumors, n (%) | 48 (80%) | 3 (5%) | 47 (78%) | 9 (15%) | >0.05 |
| Wheezing in the lungs, n(%) | 36 (60%) | 7 (12%) | 35 (58%) | 11 (22%) | >0.05 |
| Hepatomegaly, n(%) | 26 (43%) | 11 (18%) | 24 (40%) | 12 (30%) | >0.05 |
| Signs of hemostasis according to X-ray examination, n(%) | 30 (50%) | 8 (13%) | 29 (48%) | 10 (23%) | >0.05 |

We can see that there was a positive change in the NYHA functional classes of patients in both groups against the background of treatment. For example, we can observe that in sacubitril/valsartan group, 28% of patients with functional class IV according to NYHA initially had 28%, but this indicator decreased to 5% after treatment. In addition, it was observed that the patients with functional class III according to NYHA were significantly reduced in group 1, i.e. from 47% to 12% (P<0.05). On the contrary, we can observe that patients with functional class II according to NYHA have an advantage due to improvements in higher functional classes against the background of treatment (from 25% to 47%). We can observe that the functional classes of chronic heart failure improved against the background of treatment in both groups. In this group, we can observe a significant decrease in patients with NYHA functional class IV and III, and a significant increase in patients with functional class II against the background of treatment. But when the groups were compared, we could observe that the sacubitril/valsartan group had a significant effect on NYHA functional classes (R<0.05). Figure 24 shows a diagram of the change in the treatment background of the functional classes among the groups.

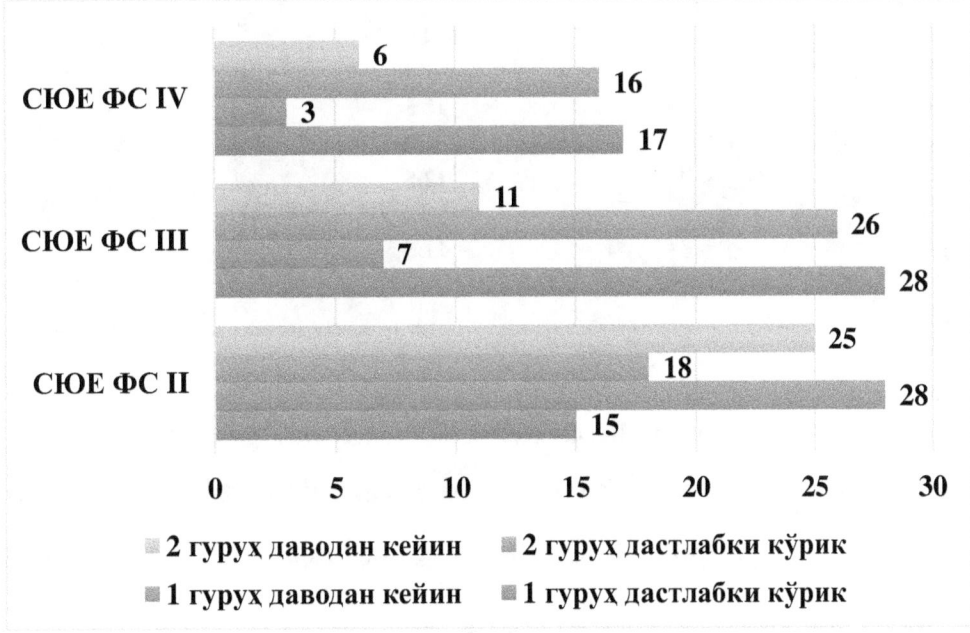

Note: Statistically significant difference when p < 0.05

**24 pictures. Functional classes between groups change in treatment background**

According to the results of the 6-minute test conducted on the patients, the average distance covered in the first examination of the patients with chronic heart failure in group 1 was 206.4±38.0 meters, and the patients' tolerance to physical exertion increased on the background of the treatment, and the average distance of the patients in this group was 379.0±48.0 meters. we can see that the distance traveled (P<0.05), while in 2 groups of patients in the initial examination, he covered a distance of 212.5±66.3 meters, and after treatment, he covered a distance of 315.0±51.0 meters (P<0.05). At the same time, the index of minute oxygen consumption in the initial examination was 12.8±6.2 ml/(kgxmin) in group 1 and reached 15.2±7.0 ml/(kgxmin) in the background of treatment (P<0.05) , and in 2 groups from 13.1±6.4 ml/(kgxmin) to 15.3±7.6 ml/(kgxmin) (P<0.05) we can observe that it has changed (Fig. 25). When the groups were compared, the 6-minute test distance was significantly higher in the sacubitril/valsartan group than in the valsartan group (P<0.05), but the oxygen demand was almost similar in both groups and no difference was observed between the groups (P> 0.05).

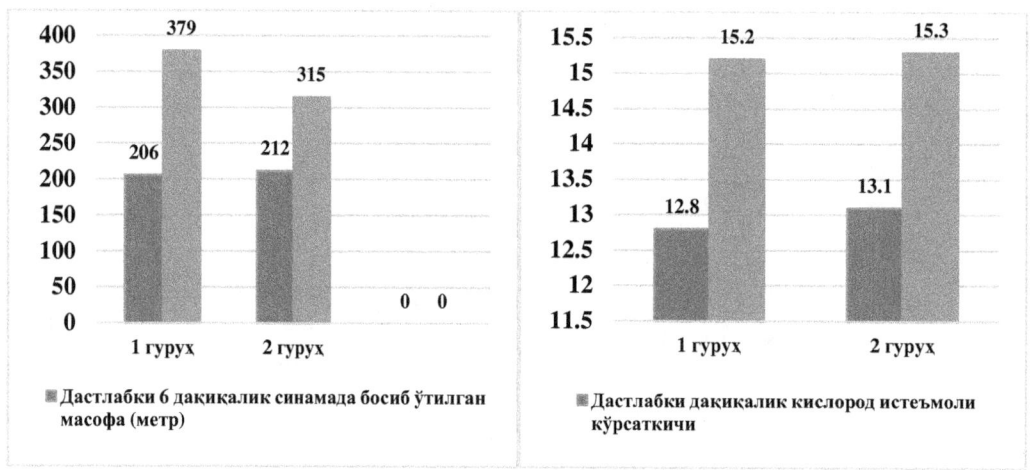

Note: Statistically significant difference when p < 0.05

**25 pictures. Average distance traveled and oxygen demand of patients in the 6-minute test in the treatment groups.**

Analyzing the hemodynamic parameters of the patients, the systolic arterial blood pressure was 129.6±19.2 mm Hg in the sacubitril/valsartan group. from 127.7±21.6 mm.cm.above. decreased by 131.6±24.5 mm.cm.sg in the valsartan group. from 129.6±23.5 mm.cm.above. was observed to decrease to Diastolic blood pressure was also observed to decrease slightly during treatment in both groups, including 78.9±12.4 mmHg in the sacubitril/valsartan group. from 77.8±12.9 mm.cm.ust. decreased by 79.0±14.1 mm.sm.sg in the valsartan group. from 77.0±14.1 mm.cm.above. was observed, but these changes were not statistically significant within groups and between groups (R>0.05). We can observe that the mean blood pressure also slightly decreased on the background of treatment in both groups, but we can see that these changes are not statistically significant (R>0.05). It can be observed that the number of heart contractions decreased from 85.4 ± 22.0 at baseline to 81.1 ± 21.6 after treatment in the sacubitril/valsartan group (R<0.05). In the Valsartan group, the number of heart contractions was reliably reduced on the background of treatment (R<0.05), but when the groups were compared, we can see that this change was not statistically significant (R>0.05; Table 28).

**28 tables**

**On the background of treatment in the groups, SAKB, DAKB and average Change of AKB and YUKS**

| Indicators | Group 1 (sacubitril/valsartan) n=60 | | 2 groups (valsartan) n=60 | | R value |
|---|---|---|---|---|---|
| | Initial indicator | Post-treatment performance | Initial indicator | Post-treatment performance | |
| SABP, mm.sm.ust. | 129.6±19.2 | 127.7±21.6 | 131.6±24.5 | 129.6±23.5 | >0.05 |
| DABP, , mm.sm.ust. | 78.9±12.4 | 77.8±12.9 | 79.0±14.1 | 77.0±14.1 | >0.05 |
| Average ABP, mm.cm.asl. | 108.8±14.4 | 107.1±14.8 | 109.1±16.2 | 106.1±15.2 | >0.05 |
| HIGH, th/min | 85.4±22.0 | 81.1±21.6* | 86.6±25.8 | 80.1±25.6* | <0.05 |

When studying NT-proBNP and BNP, which are biomarkers of chronic heart failure, we can observe that the level of NT-proBNP was 3812±1326 pg/ml at initial examination in sacubitril/valsartan group patients, and its level significantly decreased to 1835±1118 pg/ml after treatment (P <0.05). At the same time, we can observe that the amount of NT-proBNP decreased from 3612±1287 pg/ml to 2459±1154 pg/ml in the valsartan group (P<0.05). We can observe that blockers of the renin-angiotensin-aldosterone system in chronic heart failure have a positive effect on clinical manifestations of chronic heart failure as well as biomarkers. When we compared the effect of treatment on the NT-proBNP biomarker between the groups, we could see that the 1 sacubitril/valsartan group significantly reduced this biomarker compared to the valsartan group (0.012). When both groups were examined for the effect on the mean plasma concentration of BNP, a biomarker of CHF, it was found that BNP concentration changed from 512±46 pg/ml to 375±39 pg/ml in the sacubitril/valsartan group, and from 498±52 pg/ml to 412±49 pg/ml in the valsartan group. we can observe (P<0.05). When comparing the groups, we can observe that group 1 had a significant effect on BNP than group 2 (R=0.024; Table 29).

**29 tables**

**NT-proBNP, amount of BNP in groups.**

| Indicators | Group 1 (sacubitril/valsartan) n=60 | | 2 groups (valsartan) n=60 | | R value |
|---|---|---|---|---|---|
| | Initial indicator | Post-treatment performance | Initial indicator | Post-treatment performance | |
| NT-proBNP | 3812±1326 | 1835±1118* | 3612±1287 | 2459±1154* | 0.012* |
| BNP | 512±46 | 375±39* | 498±52 | 412±49* | 0.024* |

Note: *r<0.05– when compared with the phenotype of patients with reduced firing fraction;

Table 30 shows the effects of sacubitril/valsartan and valsartan groups on lipid parameters. As can be seen from the table, treatment with sacubitril/valsartan and valsartan had no significant effect on lipid parameters (P>0.05).

**30 tables**

**Quantification of lipid parameters between the initial groups.**

| Indicators | 1 group (sacubitril/valsartan) n=60 | | 2 groups (valsartan) n=60 | | R value |
|---|---|---|---|---|---|
| | Initial indicator | Post-treatment performan | Initial indicator | Post-treatment performan | |

|  |  | ce |  | ce |  |
| --- | --- | --- | --- | --- | --- |
| Total cholesterol, mmol/l | 5.1±1.7 | 3.8±1.3 | 4.9±1.9 | 3.5±1.5 | 0.125 |
| Triglyceride, mmol/l | 3.5±1.6 | 2.1±1.8 | 3.7±2.0 | 2.2±1.8 | 0.450 |
| Low-density lipoprotein cholesterol, mmol/l | 3.1±1.9 | 2.0±15 | 3.2±2.0 | 2.4±2.1 | 0.168 |
| High-density lipoprotein cholesterol, mmol/l | 1.2±0.6 | 1.1±0.9 | 1.1±0.8 | 1.0±0.7 | 0.250 |

When evaluating renal function, blood urea in the sacubitril/valsartan group decreased from 9.0±4.6 mmol/l to 8.7±4.2 mmol/l and from 8.9±4.8 mmol/l in the valsartan group. We can observe that it changed by 6±4.4 mmol/l (R>0.05). The amount of creatinine in the groups decreased from 121.0±24.4 µmol/l to 115.0±22.4 µmol/l in group 1, and from 118.0±21.9 µmol/l to 115, We can observe that it decreased to 0±20.4 µmol/l. When comparing the groups, we can observe that there was a significant effect on neither urea nor creatinine among them (R>0.05). Although the glomerular filtration rate was slightly increased in both the treatment groups, there was no significant difference between them (R>0.05). When sacubitril/valsartan and valsartan drugs were used in addition to standard treatment in patients with chronic heart failure, no significant effect of drugs on liver enzymes was observed on the background of treatment and between groups (R>0.05; Table 31).

**31 tables**

**Indicators of kidney and liver function**

| Indicators | Group 1 (sacubitril/valsartan) n=60 | | 2 groups (valsartan) n=60 | | R value |
| --- | --- | --- | --- | --- | --- |
|  | Initial | Post- | Initial | Post- |  |

|  | indicator | treatment performance | indicator | treatment performance |  |
|---|---|---|---|---|---|
| Urea, mmol/l | 9.0±4.6 | 7.8±4.2 | 8.9±4.8 | 8.0±4.4 | >0.05 |
| Creatinine, μmol/l | 121.0±24.4 | 115.0±22.4 | 118.0±21.9 | 115.0±20.4 | >0.05 |
| Ball filtration rate, ml/min, 1.73 m2 | 48.0±12.5 | 50.0±12.8 | 49.2±12.0 | 51.0±12.2 | >0.05 |
| ALT, ED/l | 22.4±9.2 | 20.4±9.8 | 25.1±7.4 | 22.0±7.2 | >0.05 |
| AST, ED/l | 24.8±14.0 | 21.2±14.9 | 26.4±12.2 | 25.4±14.2 | >0.05 |
| Bilirubin, μmol/l | 22.15±10.4 | 20.10±10.9 | 18.4±8.9 | 18.4±8.6 | >0.05 |

When evaluating general blood analysis indicators, it can be observed that there were no significant changes in the background of treatment in sacubitril/valsartan and valsartan groups (R>0.05). When the effect of groups on S-reactive protein was studied, there was a significant difference between groups (R=0.02). In particular, C-reactive protein decreased from 18.2±5.8 g/l to 11.0±5.3 g/l in the sacubitril/valsartan group, and from 20.0±8.0 g/l to 16 in the valsartan group. It can be observed that it decreased by 4±8.7 g/l (P<0.05). The effects of the sacubitril/valsartan and valsartan groups on the results of the general blood analysis are detailed in Table 32.

**32 tables**

### Initial hematological indicators of patients

| Indicators | Group 1 (sacubitril/valsartan) n=60 | | 2 groups (valsartan) n=60 | | R value |
|---|---|---|---|---|---|
|  | Initial indicator | Post-treatment performance | Initial indicator | Post-treatment performance |  |
| Hemoglobin, g/ml | 138.0±26.2 | 137.0±28.2 | 135.7±24.7 | 135.7±24.7 | 0.24 |

| Erythrocyte, 10*12/l | 4.3±2.0 | 4.2±2.4 | 4.1±1.8 | 4.0±1.2 | 0.38 |
|---|---|---|---|---|---|
| Platelet, 10*9/l | 212.0±42.5 | 219.0±46.4 | 210.4±48.9 | 214.4±45.6 | 0.27 |
| Hematocrit, % | 40.0±8.1 | 39.1±8.6 | 37.4±7.5 | 35.4±7.6 | 0.36 |
| Leukocyte, 10*9/l | 5.6±2.2 | 5.9±2.3 | 5.7±1.9 | 5.6±1.8 | 0.54 |
| CRP, g/l | 18.2±5.8 | 11.0±5.3* | 20.0±8.0 | 16.4±8.7* | 0.02** |

Note: *statistically significant difference when p < 0.05;
**p<0.05 when groups are compared.

### 3.5. Effects of 12-week treatment with sacubitril/valsartan on central and peripheral hemodynamic parameters, myocardial reserve volume and viability

Sacubitril/valsartan treatment resulted in a change in left ventricular size from 43.0±4.5 mm to 41.2±3.6 mm, while valsartan treatment resulted in a change from 42.5±4.9 mm to 40.5±4.7 mm. Although the left lobe volume decreased slightly in both groups after 3 months of treatment, the difference between them was not statistically significant (P>0.05). As a result of the treatment with sacubitril/valsartan combination, it can be observed that the left ventricular end-diastolic size decreased significantly (from 66.3±17.4 mm to 61.1±16.2 mm). In the Valsartan group, although the left ventricular end-diastolic size decreased on the background of treatment, this change was statistically insignificant (from 69.4±18.2 mm to 67.8±17.4 mm, R>0.05). When the groups were compared on the effect on the left ventricular end-diastolic size, it was observed that the effect of 1 group was significant (P=0.043). When evaluating the effect of groups on left ventricular end-systolic size, it can be observed that there was a significant change in patients in the sacubitril/valsartan group (from 54.2±14.5 mm to 50.1±14.0 mm vs. from 58.4±15.5 mm to 56,2±14.8 ha, R<0.05). Left ventricular ejection fraction significantly improved in both groups of patients (from 42.2±12.0% to 49.8±13.2% vs. from 43.1±11.9% to 47.3±14.2 %, R<0.05; 24 images). When evaluating the effect of the groups on the linear integral velocity of the left ventricular outflow, there was no significant difference between the treatment background and the groups (14.0 ± 4.6 cm to 12.6 ± 4.6 cm vs. 12.1 ± 4.4 cm to 11.7 ± by 4.3 cm, P>0.05). When evaluating the end-diastolic volume of the left ventricle, it can be observed that in the sacubitril/valsartan group this indicator changed significantly against the background of treatment (from 136.0±41.5 ml/m2 to 112.0±46.5 ml/m2 vs. 144.0±43,8 ml/m2 to 134.0±42.6 ml/m2, R<0.05; 30 tables). Although patients with chronic heart failure were treated with sacubitril/valsartan and valsartan drugs, tricuspid valve systolic excursion, tricuspid loop maximum velocity, and pulmonary artery systolic blood pressure were slightly changed, but no significant changes were observed within or between groups as a result of treatment (P>0, 05). A significant decrease in E/e' was observed on the background of treatment with sacubitril/valsartan (from 17.2±6.6 to 14.1±6.9, R>0.05), but the changes were statistically insignificant in the valsartan group (18, 3±7.0 to 17.0±7.5, P<0.05). It was found that the change in E/A was insignificant within and between groups on the background of treatment (1.6±0.5 to 1.4±0.5 vs. 1.8±0.6 to 1.5±0.4 ga, R=0.090; 30 tables). When evaluating the size of the interventricular barrier, the size of the thickness of the left ventricle, and the weight index of the left ventricle, it can be determined that there was no significant change in these indicators against the background of treatment (P>0.05). However, it can be observed that the summary index of left ventricular contractility changed differently in the groups against the background of treatment. Includingit can be observed that in the sacubitril/valsartan group, the sum index of left ventricular contractility increased from the initial 2.98±0.49 to 3.62±0.72 after 3 months of treatment (P<0.05). In the Valsartan group, although the total contractility index of the left ventricle increased, this change was statistically unreliable (P>0.05). In addition, we can observe that the sacubitril/valsartan combination significantly improved the summary index of left ventricular contractility after stress echocardiography with dobutamine compared to the valsartan group (P<0.05). Table 33 details the central and peripheral hemodynamic indicators of patients in both groups against the background of treatment.

## During observation of patients in groups echocardiographic indicators

| Indicators | Group 1 (sacubitril/valsartan) n=60 | | 2 groups (valsartan) n=60 | | R value |
|---|---|---|---|---|---|
| | Initial indicator | Post-treatment performance | Initial indicator | Post-treatment performance | |
| ChB, cm | 43.0±4.5 | 41.2±3.6 | 42.5±4.9 | 40.5±4.7 | 0.198 |
| ChQ SDO', mm | 66.3±17.4 | 61.1±16.2* | 69.4±18.2 | 67.8±17.4 | 0.043** |
| ChQ SSO', mm | 54.2±14.5 | 50.1±14.0* | 58.4±15.5 | 56.2±14.8 | 0.036** |
| ChQ firing fraction, % | 42.2±12.0 | 49.8±13.2* | 43.1±11.9 | 47.3±14.2* | 0.048** |
| Linear integral speed of the ChQ outlet, cm | 14.0±4.6 | 12.6±4.6 | 12.1±4.4 | 11.7±4.3 | 0.245 |
| ChQ SDH, ml | 136.0±41.5 | 112.0±46.5* | 144.0±43.8 | 134.0±42.6 | 0.038 |
| Assessment of tricuspid valve systolic excursion (TAPSE), mm | 18.1±4.7 | 17.8±4.9 | 15.4±4.3 | 16.2±4.6 | 0.070 |
| Maximum speed in a three-layer valve, m/s | 3.3±1.2 | 3.1±1.2 | 3.6±1.4 | 3.2±1.5 | 0.278 |
| Pulmonary artery systolic pressure, mm.sm.ust. | 18.1±6.7 | 16.2±7.1 | 19.8±6.9 | 17.9±8.1 | 0.249 |
| yes | 17.2±6.6 | 14.1±6.9* | 18.3±7.0 | 17.0±7.5 | 0.045 |
| E/A | 1.6±0.5 | 1.4±0.5 | 1.8±0.6 | 1.5±0.4 | 0.090 |
| Interventricular barrier size, mm | 1.29±0.36 | 1.25±0.39 | 1.25±0.35 | 1.21±0.38 | 0.210 |
| The size of the thickness of the left ventricle, mm | 1.28±0.38 | 1.31±0.41 | 1.19±0.33 | 1.20±0.36 | 0.218 |
| Left ventricular weight index, g/m2 | 124.4±32.5 | 122.2±35.5 | 122.4±35.0 | 122.4±37.0 | 0.172 |
| Summary index of left ventricular contractility | 2.98±0.49 | 3.62±0.72* | 2.79±0.46 | 2.85±0.51 | 0.03** |
| Summary index of left ventricular contractility after stress echocardiography | 2.2±0.69 | 3.0±0.82* | 2.3±0.68 | 2.7±0.68 | 0.04** |

| with dobutamine | | | | | |

Note: *statistically significant difference when r<0.05; **r<0.01 groups reliable difference when compared.

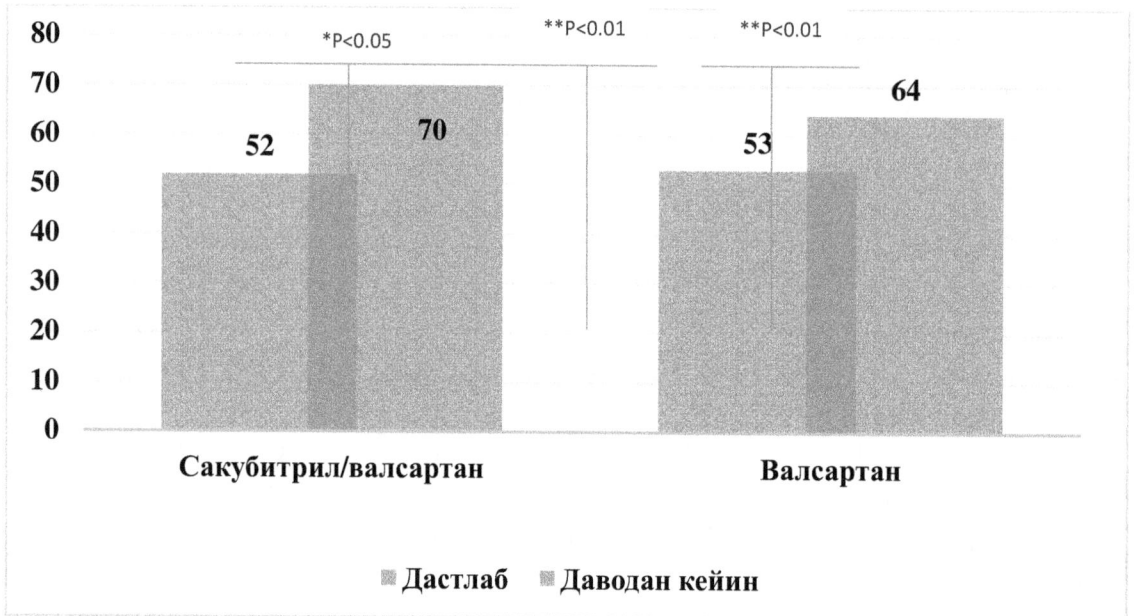

Note: *statistically significant difference when r<0.05; **r<0.01 reliable difference when comparing groups.

**26 pictures. Changes in the firing fraction in the treatment groups.**

In addition, the effects of sacubitril/valsartan and valsartan groups on ejection fraction and ejection volume on phenotypic groups of chronic heart failure separated by ejection fraction were also studied separately (Figures 26, 27, 28, 29, 30, 31, 32).

Figure 26 shows that sacubitril/valsartan combination significantly increases ejection fraction compared to valsartan combination in patients with chronic heart failure with reduced ejection fraction (EFCHF) (P<0.05). In addition, we can see that the sacubitril/valsartan combination significantly increased the firing fraction (31%) in EFCHF patients compared to the valsartan group (P<0.05; Figure 27).

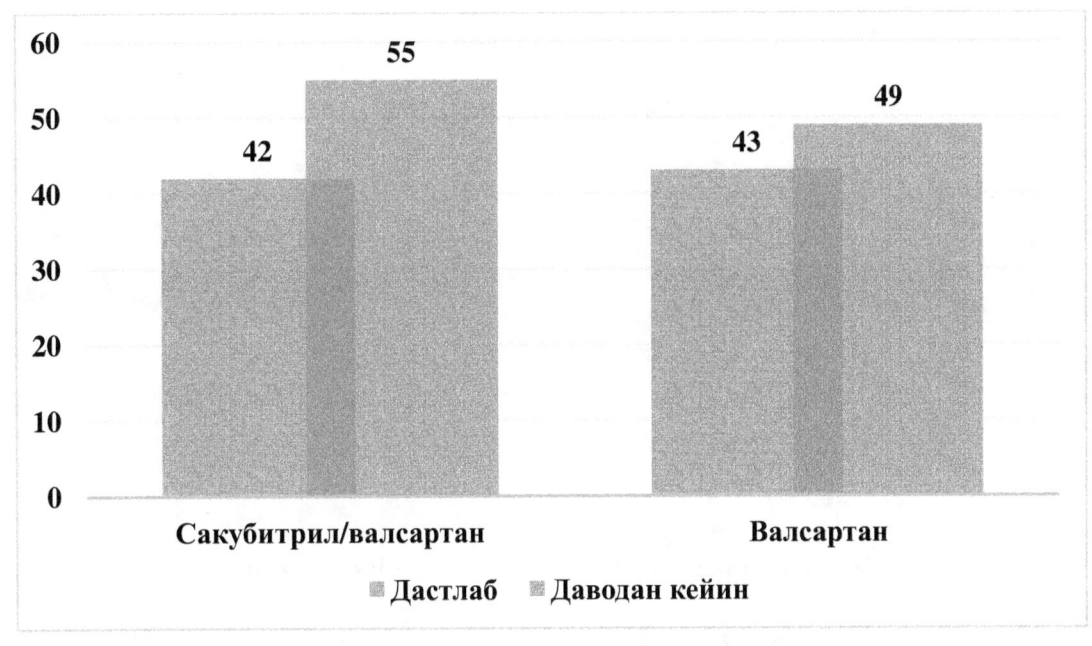

Note: Statistically significant difference when p < 0.05

**27 pictures. Effect of groups on output volume (ml) in subgroup of EFCHF patients on treatment background.**

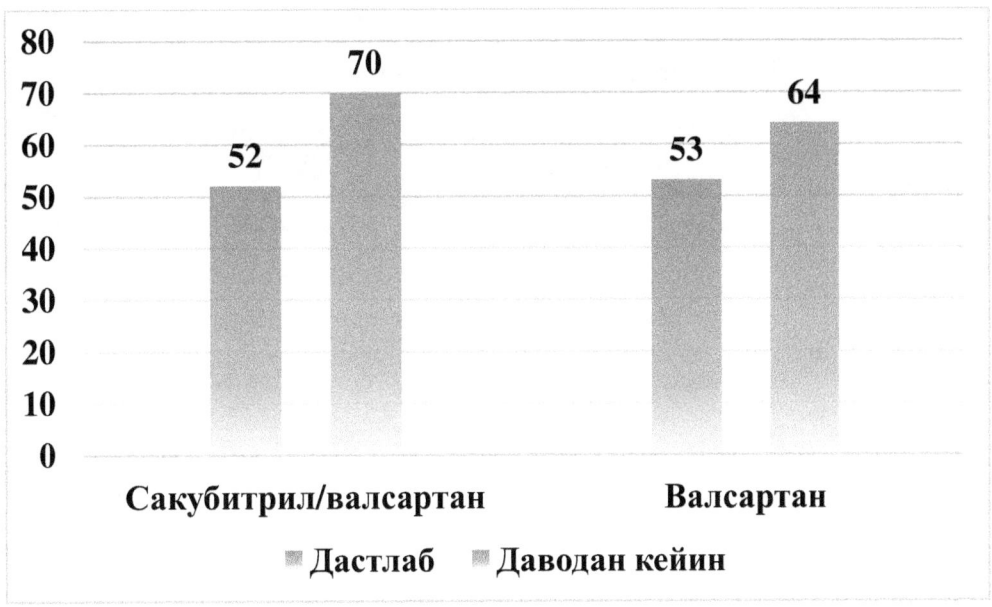

Note: Statistically significant difference when p < 0.05

**28 pictures. Effects of groups on the firing fraction (%) in the EFCHF patient subgroup on the background of treatment.**

In addition, the sacubitril/valsartan combination was superior to the valsartan group in improving ejection fraction and ejection fraction even in patients with slightly reduced ejection fraction (R<0.05; Figs. 29, 30).

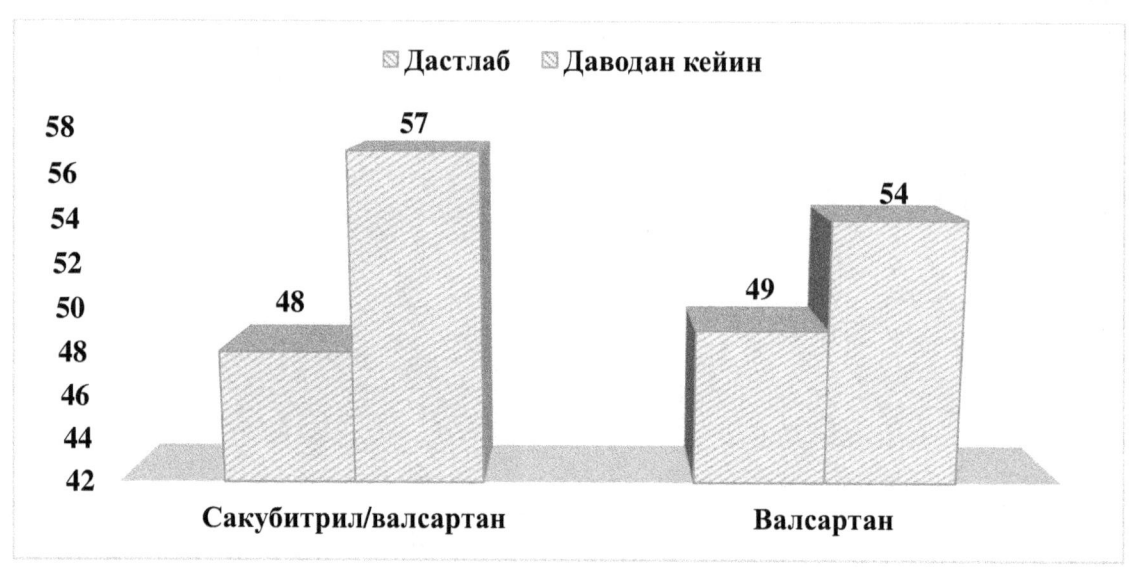

Note: Statistically significant difference when p < 0.05

**29 pictures. Effect of groups on stroke volume (ml) in subgroup of AEFCHF patients on treatment background.**

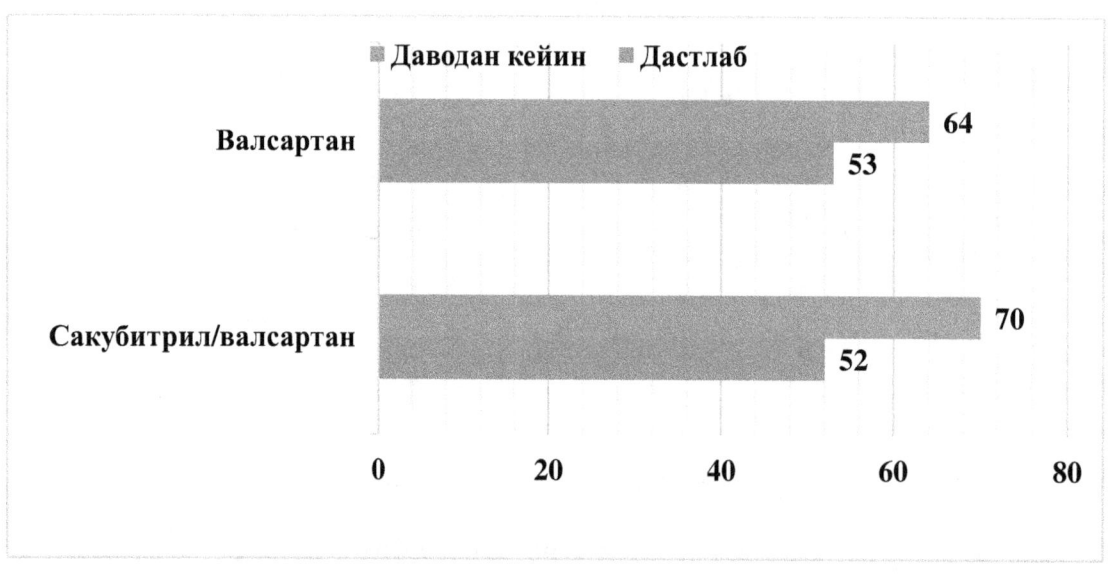

Note: Statistically significant difference when p < 0.05

**30 pictures. Effects of groups on the firing fraction (%) in the AEFCHF patient subgroup on treatment background.**

In patients with chronic heart failure with preserved ejection fraction, the sacubitril/valsartan combination and the valsartan combination showed a positive effect in improving the ejection fraction and the ejection volume after 3 months of treatment. However, these changes were not statistically significant (R>0.05). No significant change was noted when the groups were compared (R>0.05; Figure 31, Figure 32).

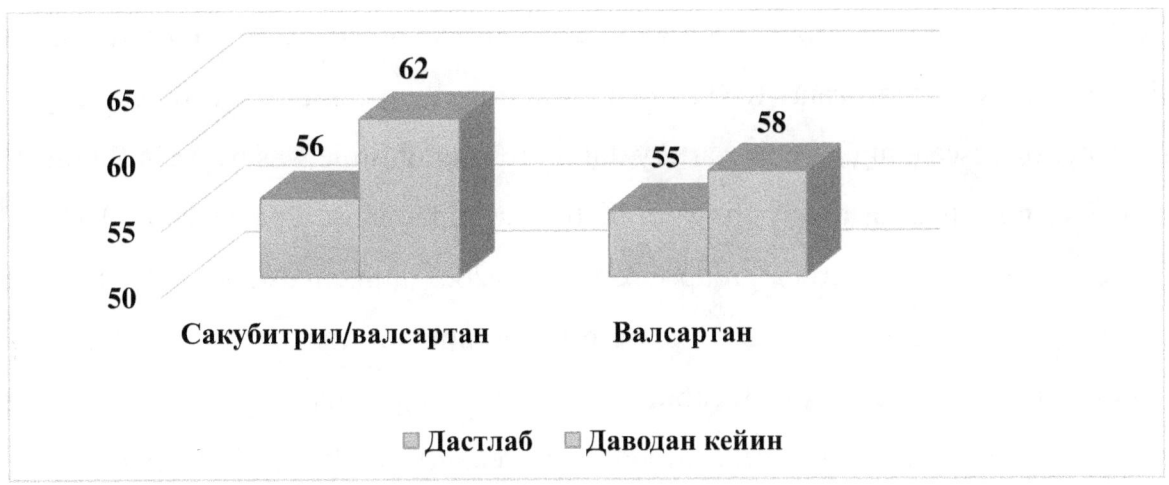

Note: Statistically significant difference when p < 0.05

**31 pictures. Effect of groups on stroke volume (ml) in subgroup of OFCCHF patients after 3 months of treatment.**

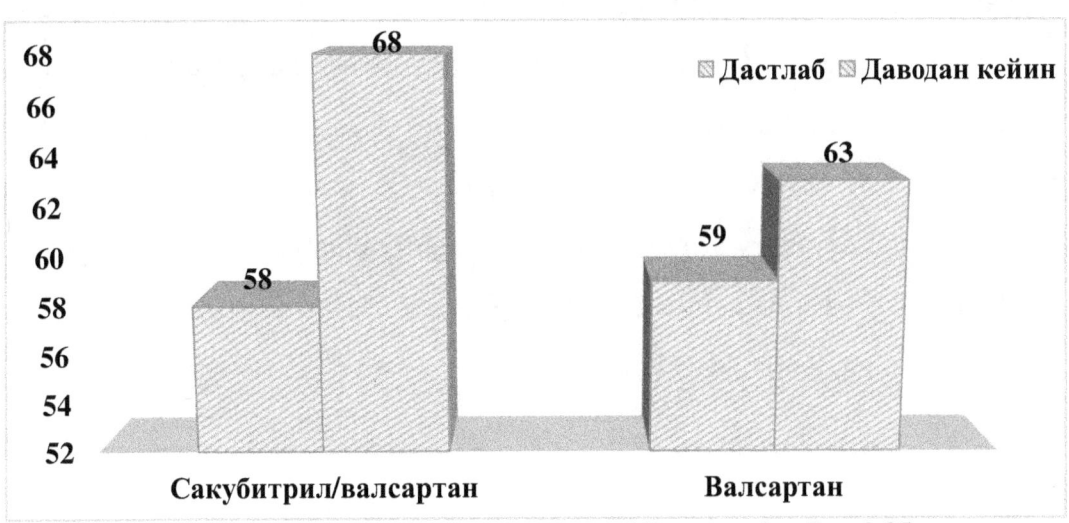

Note: Statistically significant difference when R < 0.05

**32 pictures. Effect of groups on the firing fraction (%) in the subgroup of OFCCHF patients after 3 months of treatment.**

It can be observed that significant changes were noted in the sacubitril/valsartan group when the coronary artery reserve volume of the patients was evaluated in the treatment background groups. In particular, the highest blood flow velocity in diastole during stress with the dipyridamole test of the anterior descending coronary artery was 88.0±23.0 mm.cm.sg in the sacubitril/valsartan group. from 96.0±23.0 mm.cm.ust. (P<0.05), and in the valsartan group it was 85.2±21.3 mm.cm.sg. from 89.2±21.3 mm.cm.ust. it can be observed that it increased to (P<0.05). When the groups were compared, it was noted that the changes in the first group were significant (R=0.045). In addition, the peak blood flow velocity of the anterior descending coronary artery during resting diastole was 61.5±25.0 mm Hg in the sacubitril/valsartan group. from 62.6±25.0 mm.cm.ust. changed to 59.4±20.3 mm.cm.sg. in the valsartan group. from 60.2±20.3 mm.cm.ust. slightly changed (P>0.05). We can observe that the reserve volume of the coronary artery was significantly changed in the sacubitril/valsartan group compared to the 2 groups (R=0.021). In addition, the peak blood flow velocity of the right coronary artery during stress diastole changed from 83.2±19.4 mmHg to 89.2±19.4 mmHg in the sacubitril/valsartan group, while in the valsartan group 82.8±17.9 mm.cm.ust. from 83.8±18.2 mm.cm.above. we can observe that it changed to (P>0.05). The resting diastolic peak blood flow velocity of the right coronary artery decreased from 68.0±16.0 mmHg to 69.0±16.0 mmHg in the sacubitril/valsartan group. changed to 65.2±19.4 mm.cm.sg. in the valsartan group. from 64.1±19.6 mm.cm.ust. was observed to change to (P>0.05). In addition, it can be observed that the relative reserve volume of the coronary arteries also significantly changed in the background of sacubitril/valsartan treatment in the groups (from 1.15±0.4 to 1.23±0.4 vs. from 1.11±0.6 to 1.15±0.6 ga, R=0.048; 34 tables).

## Assessment of coronary artery reserve

| Indicators | Group 1 (sacubitril/valsartan) n=60 | | 2 groups (valsartan) n=60 | | R value |
|---|---|---|---|---|---|
| | Initial indicator | Post-treatment performance | Initial indicator | Post-treatment performance | |
| VpdPNA (stress)mm.sm.ust. | 88.0±23.0 | 96.0±23.0* | 85.2±21.3 | 89.2±21.3 | 0.045 |
| VpdPNA (at rest) mm.sm.ust. | 61.5±25.0 | 62.6±25.0 | 59.4±20.3 | 60.2±20.3 | 0.120 |
| TAZ PNA | 1.4±0.4 | 1.54±0.60* | 1.4±0.35 | 1.5±0.38 | 0.021 |
| VpdPKA (stress) mm.sm.ust. | 83.2±19.4 | 89.2±19.4 | 82.8±17.9 | 83.8±18.2 | 0.069 |
| VpdPKA (at rest) mm.sm.ust. | 68.0±16.0 | 69.0±16.0 | 65.2±19.4 | 64.1±19.6 | 0.058 |
| TAZ PKA | 1.22±0.45 | 1.29±0.48* | 1.26±0.6 | 1.30±0.71 | 0.035 |
| Relative reserve volume of coronary arteries | 1.15±0.4 | 1.23±0.4* | 1.11±0.6 | 1.15±0.6 | 0.048 |

Note: statistically significant difference when *r<0.05; Vpd is the highest blood flow rate (pressure) in diastole; PNA - anterior descending artery; TAZ - reserve volume of coronary artery; PKA - right coronary artery.

As can be seen from the table above, the total and relative reserve volume of the coronary arteries were significantly increased in the sacubitril/valsartan group compared to the valsartan group, although both groups had similar results in the initial examination. In addition, the effects of sacubitril/valsartan and valsartan treatment on myocardial CHF reserve and ejection fraction phenotypes of chronic heart failure were analyzed separately. Analysis showed that the sacubitril/valsartan group improved coronary artery reserve volume in the subgroup of patients with EFCHF and AEFCHF of CHF, but the change in ejection fraction in OFCCHF was slightly improved in both groups, with no significant difference between groups (Figures 33,34,35).

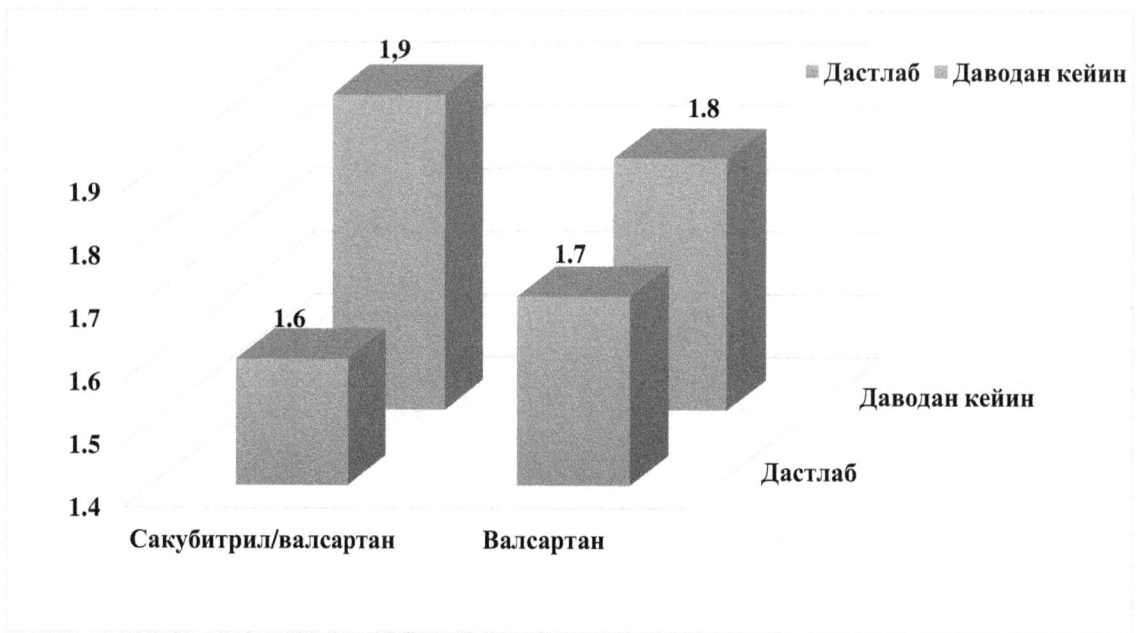

Note: Statistically significant difference when $p < 0.05$

**33 pictures. EFCHF changes in reserve volume of coronary arteries**

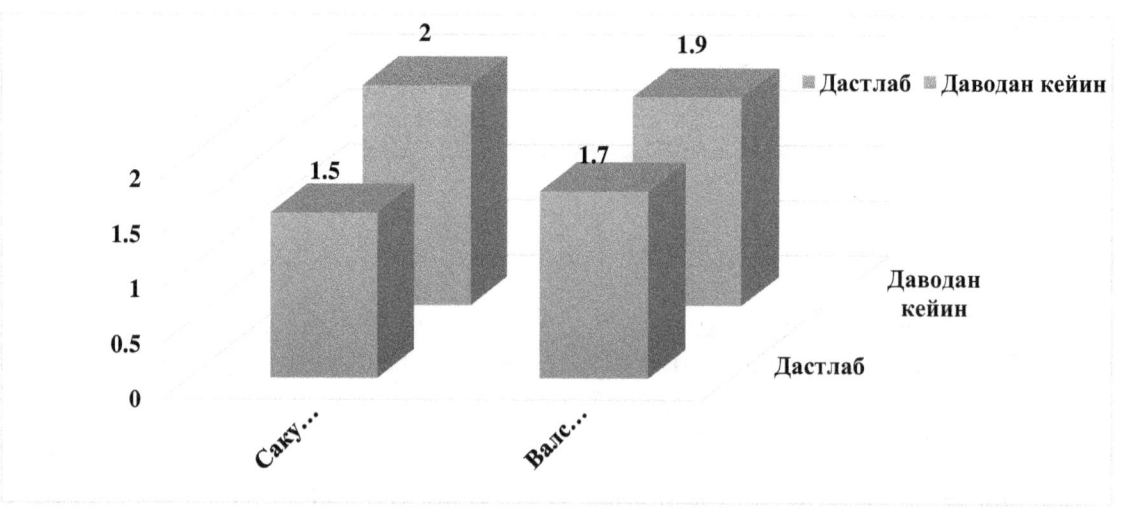

Note: Statistically significant difference when $p < 0.05$

**34 pictures. AEFCHF changes in reserve volume of coronary arteries**

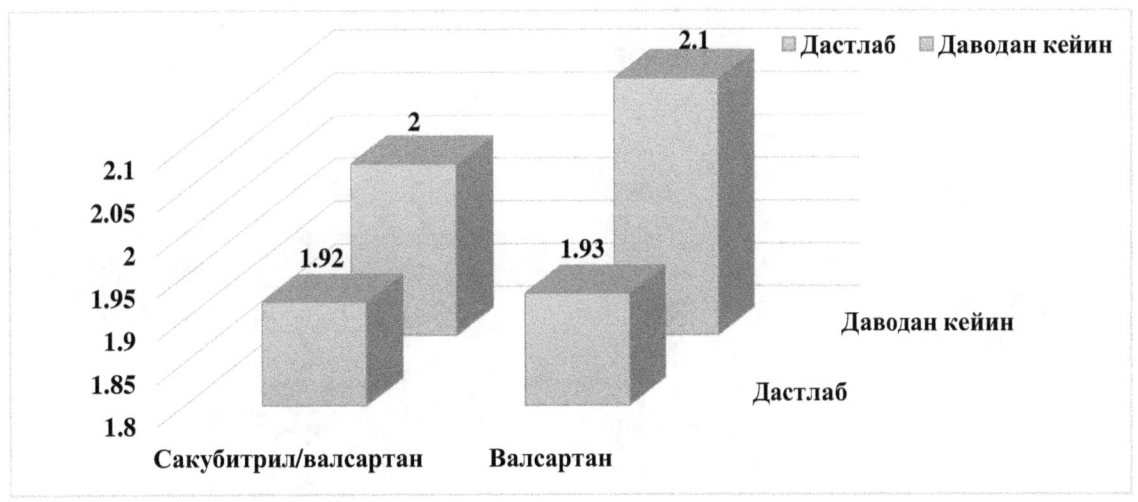

Note: Statistically significant difference when p < 0.05

**35 pictures. OfCHF changes in the reserve volume of coronary arteries**

The effect of the sacubitril/valsartan combination on coronary artery reserve volume suggests a specific advantage of this agent in patients with chronic heart failure of ischemic etiology. The improvement of the coronary artery reserve volume of this drug in CHF in EFCHF and AEFCHF shows the superiority of sacubitril/valsartan, and in patients with OFCCHF, both groups are effective in improving the volume of coronary artery reserve. No significant difference was observed between men and women in all forms of chronic heart failure (R>0.05) when a separate analysis was conducted by gender.

Based on the conducted research and obtained results, an algorithm for diagnosis and treatment of CHF was developed (Fig. 36).

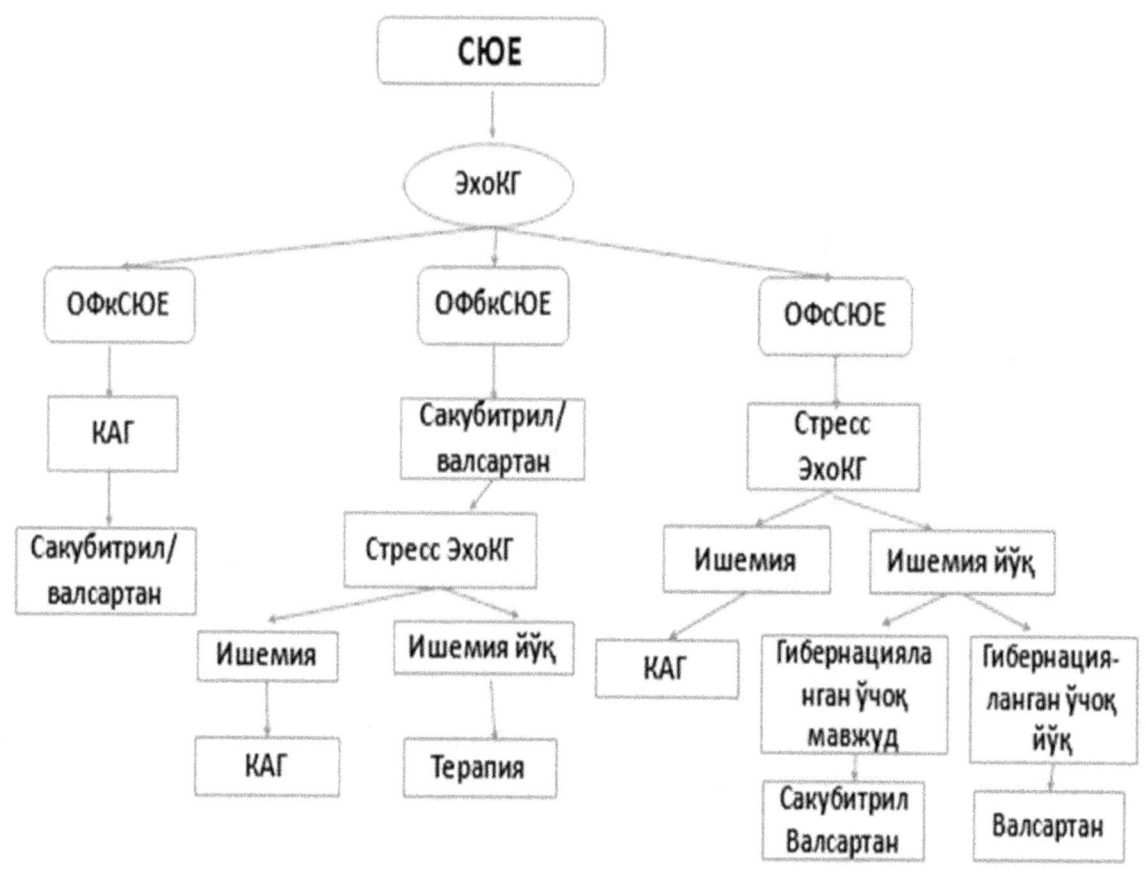

**36 pictures. Algorithm for diagnosis and treatment of patients with CHF.**

## LIST OF REFERENCES USED

1. Alyavi B.A., Muminov Sh.K.. Vliyanie sakubitrila na process stanovleniya i progressirovaniya XBP u bolnyx IBS // Evraziyskiy vestnik pediatrii. — 2020; 4 (7): 32-39

2. Galochkin S.A, Lukina O.I., Meray I.A, Villevalde S.V., Kobalava J.D. Experience of hospital initiation of sacubitril/valsartan in patients after episodic decompensation of cardiac insufficiency. Cardiology. 2018. T58. No. S5. C.60–64.

3. Kobalava J.D., Villevalde S.V., Lukina O.I. Breakthrough and treatment of patients with heart failure with low fractional vibration: the clinical significance of the PARADIGM-HF study. Cardiology. 2017. No. 2. S. 76–82

4. Kobalava J.D., Villevalde S.V., Meray I.A, Lukina O.I. Effect of sacubitril/valsartan on natriuresis, diuresis and level of arterial pressure in patients with arterial hypertension. Rational pharmacotherapy and cardiology. 2017. T13. No. 3. S 370–377.

5. Kobalava J.D., Villevalde S.V., Meray I.A, Shkolnikova E.E., Lukina O.I. Effects of sacubitril/valsartan on parameters of arterial rigidity and left-ventricular-arterial coupling in patients with heart failure and low fractional vibration. Ratsionalnaya pharmacoterapiya v kardiologii. 2018. T14. No. 2. S 210–216.

6. Kopeva K.V. Autoreferat na temu Rol GPG 2 v prognozirovanii razvitiya devechnososudistyx oslojnenii i vyborestrategii therapyi u bolnykh kronicheskoy koredechnoi destatochnostyu ishemicheskogo genesis s i bez narusheniy glyvodnogo mena// 2018, Tomsk

7. Mareev V.Yu., Fomin I.V., Ageev F.T. i dr. Klinicheskie rekomendatsii OSSN – RKO – RNMOT. Heart failure: chronic (XSN) and acute decompensated (ODSN). Diagnostics, prevention and treatment. Cardiology. 2018. T. 58(6S). S. 8–158.

8. Shlyakhto E.V. "Cardiology" National leadership 2 oe izdanie Moskva izdatelskaya group "GEOTAR-Media" 2019, str. 628-689

9. Iqbol Adilova, Gulnoza Akbarova "Effective effect of sacubitril/valsartan on

left ventricular systolic function in heart failure and low fractional patients" - Society and innovations Special IsCHF - 4 (2021) / ISSN 2181-1415

10. Tashkenbaeva NF, TrigulovaR.Kh., Khalikova AO, MukhtarovaSh.Sh. Mechanisms of formation of heart dysfunction and the application of sakubutri/valsartan in diabetes mellitus. Journal of cardiorespiratory research. 2021, vol 2., isCHF 2, pp 34-38.

11. Braunwald E. The war against heart failure: the Lancet lecture. Lancet. 2015 Feb 28;385(9970):812–24.

12. GBD 2017 DALYs and HALE Collaborators. Global, regional, and national disability-adjusted life-years (DALYs) for 359 diseases and injuries and healthy life expectancy (HALE) for 195 countries and territories, 1990-2017: a systematic analysis for the Global Burden of Disease Study 2017. Lancet 2018;392:1859-922.

13. Benjamin EJ, Muntner P, Alonso A, et al. Heart Disease and Stroke Statistics-2019 Update: A Report From the American Heart Association. Circulation 2019;139:e56-528.

14. Ionescu RF, Cretoiu SM. MicroRNAs as monitoring markers for right-sided heart failure and congestive hepatopathy. J Med Life. 2021 Mar-Apr;14(2):142-147. doi: 10.25122/jml-2021-0071. PMID: 34104236; PMCID: PMC8169151.

15. P. Ponikowski, AA Voors, SD Anker et al., "2016 ESC Guidelines for the diagnosis and treatment of acute and chronic heart failure," European Heart Journal, vol. 37, no. 27, pp. 2129–2200, 2016.

16. Mentz RJ, O'Connor CM. Pathophysiology and clinical evaluation of acute heart failure. Nat Rev Cardiol. (2016) 13:28–35. doi: 10.1038/nrcardio.2015.134

17. Savarese G, Lund LH. Global Public Health Burden of Heart Failure. Cardiac Failure Reviews 2017;3:7-11.

18. Seferovic PM, Ponikowski P, Anker SD, Bauersachs J, Chioncel O, Cleland JGF, de Boer RA, Drexel H, Ben Gal T, Hill L, Jaarsma T, Jankowska EA, Anker MS, Lainscak M, Lewis BS, McDonagh T, Metra M, Milicic D, Mullens W, Piepoli MF, Rosano G, Ruschitzka F, Volterrani M, Voors AA, Filippatos G, Coats AJS (2019) Clinical practice update on heart failure 2019: pharmacotherapy, procedures,

devices and patient management. An expert consensus meeting report of the Heart Failure Association of the European Society of Cardiology. Eur J Heart Fail 21:1169–1186

19. Filippatos G, Farmakis D, Bistola V, Karavidas A, Mebazaa A, Maggioni AP, Parissis J (2014) Temporal trends in epidemiology, clinical presentation and management of acute heart failure: results from the Greek cohorts of the Acute Heart Failure Global Registry of Standard Treatment and the European Society of Cardiology Heart Failure pilot survey. Eur Heart J Acute Cardiovasc Care.

20. Kurmani S, Squire I. Acute heart failure: definition, classification and epidemiology. Curr Heart Fail Rep. 2017;14(5):385–92.

21. Andronic AA, Mihaila S, Cinteza M. Heart Failure with mid-range ejection fraction – a new category of heart failure or still a gray zone. Maedica (Bucur) 2016;11:320–4.

22. GBD 2016 Disease and Injury Incidence and Prevalence Collaborators, "Global, regional, and national incidence, prevalence, and years lived with disability for 328 diseases and injuries for 195 countries, 1990-2016: a systematic analysis for the Global Burden of Disease Study 2016 ," Lancet, vol. 390, no. 10100, pp. 1211–1259, 2017.

23. GBD 2013 Mortality and Causes of Death Collaborators. Global, regional, and national age-sex specific all-cause and cause-specific mortality for 240 causes of death, 1990-2013: a systematic analysis for the Global Burden of Disease Study 2013. Lancet. (2015) 385:117–71. doi: 10.1016/S0140-6736(14)61682-2

24. Benjamin EJ, Blaha MJ, Chiuve SE, et al. American Heart Association Statistics Committee and Stroke Statistics Subcommittee. Heart disease and stroke statistics – 2017 update: a report from the American Heart Association. Circulation 2017;135:e146–603.

25. Dokainish H, Teo K, Zhu J, et al. Global mortality variations in patients with heart failure: results from the International Congestive Heart Failure (INTER-CHF) prospective cohort study. Lancet Glob Health 2017;5:e665-72.

26. MacDonald MR, Tay WT, Teng TK, et al. Regional Variation of Mortality

in Heart Failure With Reduced and Preserved Ejection Fraction Across Asia: Outcomes in the ASIAN-HF Registry. J Am Heart Assoc 2020;9:e012199.

27. Hao G, Wang X, Chen Z, Zhang L, Zhang Y, Wei B, et al. Prevalence of heart failure and left ventricular dysfunction in China: the China hypertension survey, 2012-2015. Eur J Heart Failure. (2019) 21:1329–37. doi: 10.1002/ejhf.1629

28. Gedela M, Khan M, Jonsson O. Heart Failure. SD Med. 2015 Sep;68(9):403-5, 407-9.

29. Waikar SS, Mount DB, Curhan GC. Mortality after hospitalization with mild, moderate, and severe hyponatremia. Am J Med. 2009 Sep;122(9):857–65.

30. Ponikowski P, Voors AA, Anker SD, et al. 2016 ESC Guidelines for the diagnosis and treatment of acute and chronic heart failure: The Task Force for the diagnosis and treatment of acute and chronic heart failure of the European Society of Cardiology (ESC). Eur J Heart Fail 2016;18:891-975.

31. Fomin I. V. Ageev F.T. i saavt. Epidemiology of chronic heart failure in the Russian Federation. V kn.: Chronic heart failure. M.: GEOTAR-Media, 2010: 7-77.

32. Lawson CA, Zaccardi F, Squire I, et al. 20-Year Trends in Cause-Specific Heart Failure Outcomes by Sex, Socioeconomic Status, and Place of Diagnosis: A Population-Based Study. Lancet Public Health 2019;4:e406-20.

33. Coronel, R., de Groot, JR, & van Lieshout, JJ (2001). Defining heart failure. Cardiovascular research, 50(3), 419–422.

34. Ionescu RF, Cretoiu SM. MicroRNAs as monitoring markers for right-sided heart failure and congestive hepatopathy. J Med Life. 2021 Mar-Apr;14(2):142-147.

35. Tan LB, Williams SG, Tan DK et al. So many definitions of heart failure: are they all universally valid? A critical appraisal. Expert Rev Cardiovasc Ther. 2010;8:217–228.

36. Metra, M., & Teerlink, JR (2017). Heart failure. Lancet (London, England), 390(10106), 1981–1995.

37. Yancy, CW, Jessup, M., Bozkurt, B., Butler, J., Casey, DE, Jr, Colvin, MM, Drazner, MH, Filippatos, GS, Fonarow, GC, Givertz, MM, Hollenberg, SM, Lindenfeld. , J., Masoudi, FA, McBride, PE, Peterson, PN, Stevenson, LW, &

Westlake, C. (2017). 2017 ACC/AHA/HFCA Focused Update of the 2013 ACCF/AHA Guideline for the Management of Heart Failure: A Report of the American College of Cardiology/American Heart Association Task Force on Clinical Practice Guidelines and the Heart Failure Society of America. Circulation, 136(6), e137–e161.

38. Pfeffer, MA, Shah, AM, & Borlaug, BA (2019). Heart Failure With Preserved Ejection Fraction In Perspective. Circulation research, 124(11), 1598–1617.

39. Crespo-Leiro, MG, Metra, M., Lund, LH, Milicic, D., Costanzo, MR, Filippatos, G., GustaFCson, F., Tsui, S., Barge-Caballero, E., De Jonge, N. ., Frigerio, M., Hamdan, R., Hasin, T., Hülsmann, M., Nalbantgil, S., Potena, L., Bauersachs, J., Gkouziouta, A., Ruhparwar, A., Ristic, AD, … Ruschitzka, F. (2018). Advanced heart failure: a position statement of the Heart Failure Association of the European Society of Cardiology. European journal of heart failure, 20(11), 1505–1535.

40. Snipelisky, D., Chaudhry, SP, & Stewart, GC (2019). The Many Faces of Heart Failure. Cardiac electrophysiology clinics, 11(1), 11–20.

41. Brady, C., Ministeri, M., Kempny, A., Alonso-Gonzalez, R., Swan, L., Webing, A., Diller, GP, Gatzoulis, MA, & Dimopoulos, K. (2018). New York Heart Association (NYHA) classification in adults with congenital heart disease: relation to objective measures of exercise and outcome. European heart journal. Quality of care & clinical outcomes, 4(1), 51–58.

42. Van der Meer, P., Gaggin, HK, & Dec, GW (2019). ACC/AHA Versus ESC Guidelines on Heart Failure: JACC Guideline Comparison. Journal of the American College of Cardiology, 73(21), 2756–2768.

43. Leri A, Rota M, Pasqualini FC, Goichberg P, Anversa P. Origin of cardiomyocytes in the adult heart. Circ Res. 2015 Jan 2; 116(1):150-66.

44. Kumar V, Abbas AK, Fausto N. Robbins and Cotran Pathologic basis of disease. Elsevier Saunders; 2005.

45. Bray MA, Sheehy SP, Parker KK. Sarcomere alignment is regulated by

myocyte shape. Cell Motile Cytoskeleton. 2008 Aug; 65(8):641-51.

46. Sanger JW, Ayoob JC, Chowrashi P, Zurawski D, Sanger JM. Assembly of myofibrils in cardiac muscle cells. Adv Exp Med Biol. 2000; 481():89-102; discussion 103-5.

47. Opie LH. Heart Physiology: From Cell to Circulation. Lippincott Williams & Wilkins, 2003.

48. Li F, Wang X, Yi XP, Gerdes AM. Structural basis of ventricular remodeling: role of the myocyte. Curr Heart Fail Rep. 2004 Apr-May; 1(1):5-8.

49. Russell B, Curtis MW, Koshman YE, Samarel AM. Mechanical stress-induced sarcomere assembly for cardiac muscle growth in length and width. J Mol Cell Cardiol. 2010 May; 48(5):817-23.

50. Frank O. Zur Dynamik des Herzmuskels. J. Biol 32 (1895) 370–447. Translation from German: Chapman CP, Wasserman EB. On the dynamics of cardiac muscle. Am. Heart J 58 (1959) 282–317.

51. Holubarsch C, Ruf T, Goldstein DJ, Ashton RC, Nickl W, Pieske B, Pioch K, Lüdemann J, Wiesner S, Hasenfuss G, Posival H, Just H, Burkhoff D. Existence of the Frank-Starling mechanism in the failing human heart. Investigations on the organ, CHF, and sarcomere levels. Circulation. 1996 Aug 15; 94(4):683-9.

52. Opie LH, Commerford PJ, Gersh BJ, Pfeffer MA. Controversies in ventricular remodeling. Lancet. 2006 Jan 28; 367(9507):356-67.

53. Genet M, Lee LC, Baillargeon B, Guccione JM, Kuhl E. Modeling Pathologies of Diastolic and Systolic Heart Failure. Ann Biomed Eng. 2016 Jan; 44(1):112-27.

54. Anand IS, Latini R, Florea VG, Kuskowski MA, Rector T, Masson S, Signorini S, Mocarelli P, Hester A, Glazer R, Cohn JN. C-reactive protein in heart failure: prognostic value and the effect of valsartan. Circulation 2005;112:1428–1434.

55. Swirski FK, Nahrendorf M. Leukocyte behavior in atherosclerosis, myocardial infarction, and heart failure. Science 2013;339:161–166.

56. Mortensen RM. Immune cell modulation of cardiac remodeling. Circulation

2012;125:1597–1600.

57. Liu L, Wang Y, Cao Z, Wang M, Liu X, Gao T, Hu Q, Yuan W, Lin L. Up-regulated TLR4 in cardiomyocytes exacerbates heart failure after long-term myocardial infarction. J Cell Mol Med 2015;19:2728–2740.

58. Frangogiannis NG, Singh M, Singh K, Rivera L, Brecken R, Bradshaw A. The extracellular matrix in myocardial injury, repair, and remodeling. J Clin Invest 2017;127:1600–1612.

59. Coles B, Fielding CA, Rose-John S, Scheller J, Jones SA, O'Donnell VB. Classic interleukin-6 receptor signaling and interleukin-6 trans-signaling differentially control angiotensin II-dependent hypertension, cardiac signal transducer and activator of transcription-3 activation, and vascular hypertrophy in vivo. Am J Pathol 2007;171:315–325.

60. Zipes DP. Heart-brain interactions in cardiac arrhythmias: role of the autonomic nervous system. Cleve Clin J Med. 2008 Mar; 75 Suppl 2():S94-6.

61. Pierpont GL, DeMaster EG, Reynolds S, Pederson J, Cohn JN. Ventricular myocardial catecholamines in primates. J Lab Clin Med. 1985 Aug; 106(2):205-10.

62. Armor JA. Cardiac neuronal hierarchy in health and disease. Am J Physiol Regul Integr Comp Physiol. 2004 Aug; 287(2):R262-71.

63. Aggarwal A, Esler MD, Lambert GW, Hastings J, Johnston L, Kaye DM. Norepinephrine turnover is increased in suprabulbar subcortical brain regions and is related to whole-body sympathetic activity in human heart failure. Circulation. 2002 Mar 5; 105(9):1031-3.

64. Philipp M, Hein L. Adrenergic receptor knockout mice: distinct functions of 9 receptor subtypes. Pharmacol Ther. 2004 Jean; 101(1):65-74.

65. Dzau VJ, Colucci WS, Hollenberg NK, Williams GH. Relation of the renin-angiotensin-aldosterone system to clinical state in congestive heart failure. Circulation. 1981 Mar; 63(3):645-51.

66. Pepper GS, Lee RW. Sympathetic activation in heart failure and its treatment with beta-blockade. Arch Intern Med. 1999 Feb 8; 159(3):225-34.

67. Morris MJ, Cox HS, Lambert GW, Kaye DM, Jennings GL, Meredith IT,

Esler MD. Region-specific neuropeptide Y overflows at rest and during sympathetic activation in humans. Hypertension. 1997 Jean; 29(1 Pt 1):137-43.

68. Hogg K, McMurray J. Neurohumoral pathways in heart failure with preserved systolic function. Prog Cardiovasc Dis. 2005 May-June; 47(6):357-66.

69. Abassi Z, Karram T, Ellaham S, Winaver J, Hoffman A. Implications of the natriuretic peptide system in the pathogenesis of heart failure: diagnostic and therapeutic importance. PharmacolTher2004;102:223–241.

70. Ponikowski P, Voors AA, Anker SD, Bueno H, Cleland JG, Coats AJ, Falk V, González Juanatey JR, Harjola VP, Jankowska EA, Jessup M, Linde C, Nihoyannopoulos P, Parissis JT, Pieske B, Riley JP, Rosano GM, Ruilope LM, Ruschitzka F, Rutten FH, van der Meer P. 2016 ESC Guidelines for the diagnosis and treatment of acute and chronic heart failure: The Task Force for the diagnosis and treatment of acute and chronic heart failure of the European Society of Cardiology (ESC). Developed with the special contribution of the Heart Failure Association (HFA) of the ESC. Eur J Heart Fail 2016;18:891–975.

71. Volpe M, Carnovali M, Mastromarino V. The natriuretic peptides system in the pathophysiology of heart failure: from molecular basis to treatment. Clin Sci (Lond) 2016;130:57–77.

72. Volpe M, Rubattu S, Burnett J Jr. Natriuretic peptides in cardiovascular diseases: current use and perspectives. Eur Heart J 2014;35:419–425.

73. Kerkelä R, Ulvila J, Magga J. Natriuretic peptides in the regulation of cardiovascular physiology and metabolic events. J Am Heart Assoc 2015;4:e002423.

74. McMurray JJ, Adamopoulos S, Anker SD, Auricchio A, Bohm M, Dickstein K, Falk V, Filippatos G, Fonseca C, Gomez-Sanchez MA, Jaarsma T, Kober L, Lip GY, Maggioni AP, Parkhomenko A, Pieske BM, Popescu BA, Ronnevik PK, Rutten FH, Schwitter J, Seferovic P, Stepinska J, Trindade PT, Voors AA, Zannad F, Zeiher A, Task Force for the Diagnosis and Treatment of Acute and Chronic Heart Failure 2012 of the European Society of Cardiology , Bach JJ, Baumgartner H, Ceconi C, Dean W, Deaton C, Fagard R, Funck-Brentano C, Hasdai D, Hoes A, Kirchhof P, Knuuti J, Kohl P, McDonagh T, Moulin C, Popescu BA, Reiner Z , SechtemU, Sirnes

PA, Tendera M, Torbicki A, Vahanian A, Windecker S, McDonagh T, Sechtem U, Bonet LA, Avraamides P, Ben Lamin HA, Brignole M, Coca A, Cowburn P, Dargie H, Elliott P, Flachskampf FA, Guida GF, Hardman S, Iung B, Merkely B, Mueller C, Nanas JN, Nielsen OW, Orn S, Parissis JT, Ponikowski P, ESC Committee for Practice Guidelines. ESC guidelines for the diagnosis and treatment of acute and chronic heart failure 2012: The Task Force for the Diagnosis and Treatment of Acute and Chronic Heart Failure 2012 of the European Society of Cardiology. Developed in collaboration with the Heart Failure Association (HFA) of the ESC. Eur J Heart Fail 2012;14:803–869.

75. Diez M, Talavera ML, Conde DG, Campos R, Acosta A, Trivi MS. High-sensitivity troponin is associated with high risk clinical profile and outcome in acute heart failure. Cardiol J. 2016;23(1):78-83.

76. Isabell Jan, Christine S. Börschel, Johannes T. Neumann, Ngoc A. Sprünker, Natalia Makarova, Jukka Contto, Kari Kuulasmaa, VeikkoSalomaa, Christina Magnussen, LiciaIacoviello, Augusto Di Castelnuovo, Simona Costanzo, Allan Linneberg, Stefan Söderberg, Tanja Zeller, Francisco M. Ojeda-Echevarria, Stefan Blankenberg, and Dirk Westermann. High-Sensitivity Cardiac Troponin I Levels and Prediction of Heart Failure: Results From the BiomarCaRE Consortium. J Am Coll Cardiol HF. 2020 May, 8(5) 401–411.

77. Liuzzo G, Santamaria M, Biasucci LM, Narducci M, Colafrancesco V, Porto A, Brugaletta S, Pinnelli M, Rizzello V, Maseri A, Crea F. Persistent activation of nuclear factor kappa-B signaling pathway in patients with unstable angina and elevated levels of C-reactive protein evidence for a direct proinflammatory effect of azide and lipopolysaccharide-free C-reactive protein on human monocytes via nuclear factor kappa-B activation. J Am Coll Cardiol. 2007 Jan 16; 49(2):185-94.

78. ELSTER SK, BRAUNWALD E, WOOD HF. A study of C-reactive protein in the serum of patients with congestive heart failure. Am Heart J. 1956 Apr; 51(4):533-41.

79. Kaneko K, Kanda T, Yamauchi Y, Hasegawa A, Iwasaki T, Arai M, Suzuki T, Kobayashi I, Nagai R C-reactive protein in dilated cardiomyopathy.Cardiology.

1999; 91(4):215-9.

80. Anand IS, Latini R, Florea VG, Kuskowski MA, Rector T, Masson S, Signorini S, Mocarelli P, Hester A, Glazer R, Cohn JN, Val-HeFT Investigators. C-reactive protein in heart failure: prognostic value and the effect of valsartan. Circulation. 2005 Sep 6; 112(10):1428-34.

81. Lamblin N, Mouquet F, Hennache B, Dagorn J, Susen S, Bauters C, de Groote P. High-sensitivity C-reactive protein: potential adjunct for risk stratification in patients with stable congestive heart failure. Eur Heart J. 2005 Nov; 26(21):2245-50.

82. Windram JD, Loh PH, Rigby AS, Hanning I, Clark AL, Cleland JG. Relationship of high-sensitivity C-reactive protein to prognosis and other prognostic markers in outpatients with heart failure. Am Heart J. 2007 Jun; 153(6):1048-55.

83. Dunlay SM, Gerber Y, Weston SA, Killian JM, Redfield MM, Roger VL. Prognostic value of biomarkers in heart failure: application of novel methods in the community. Circ Heart Fail. 2009 Sep; 2(5):393-400.

84. Galijasevic S, Saed GM, Diamond MP, Abu-Soud HM. Myeloperoxidase up-regulates the catalytic activity of inducible nitric oxide synthase by preventing nitric oxide feedback inhibition. Proc Natl Acad Sci U S A. 2003 Dec 9; 100(25):14766-71.

85. Zhang R, Brennan ML, Fu X, Aviles RJ, Pearce GL, Penn MS, Topol EJ, Sprecher DL, Hazen SL. Association between myeloperoxidase levels and risk of coronary artery disease. JAMA. 2001 Nov 7; 286(17):2136-42.

86. Tang WH, Brennan ML, Philip K, Tong W, Mann S, Van Lente F, Hazen SL. Plasma myeloperoxidase levels in patients with chronic heart failure. Am J Cardiol. 2006 Sep 15; 98(6):796-9.

87. Tang WH, Katz R, Brennan ML, Aviles RJ, Tracy RP, Psaty BM, Hazen SL Usefulness of myeloperoxidase levels in healthy elderly subjects to predict risk of developing heart failure. Am J Cardiol. 2009 May 1; 103(9):1269-74.

88. Ng LL, Pathick B, Loke IW, Squire IB, Davies JE. Myeloperoxidase and C-reactive protein augment the specificity of B-type natriuretic peptide in community

screening for systolic heart failure. Am Heart J. 2006 Jul; 152(1):94-101.

89. Tang WH, Shrestha K, Troughton RW, Borowski AG, Klein AL. Integrating plasma high-sensitivity C-reactive protein and myeloperoxidase for risk prediction in chronic systolic heart failure. Congestive Heart Failure. 2011 May-June; 17(3):105-9.

90. Kakkar R, Lee RT. The IL-33/GPG 2 pathway: therapeutic target and novel biomarker. Nat Rev Drug Discov. 2008 Oct; 7(10):827-40.

91. Sanada S, Hakuno D, Higgins LJ, Schreiter ER, McKenzie AN, Lee RT. IL-33 and GPG 2 comprise a critical biomechanically induced and cardioprotective signaling system. J Clin Invest. 2007 Wool; 117(6):1538-49.

92. Pascual-Figal DA, Pérez-Martínez MT, Asensio-Lopez MC, Sanchez-Más J, García-García ME, Martinez CM, Lencina M, Jara R, Januzzi JL, Lax A. Pulmonary Production of Soluble GPG 2 in Heart Failure. Circ Heart Fail. 2018 Dec; 11(12):e005488.

93. Parikh RH, Seliger SL, Christenson R, Gottdiener JS, Psaty BM, deFilippi CR. Soluble GPG 2 for Prediction of Heart Failure and Cardiovascular Death in an Elderly, Community-Dwelling Population. J Am Heart Assoc. 2016 Aug 1; 5(8).

94. Weinberg EO, Shimpo M, Hurwitz S, Tominaga S, Rouleau JL, Lee RT. Identification of serum soluble GPG 2 receptor as a novel heart failure biomarker. Circulation. 2003 Feb 11; 107(5):721-6.

95. Felker GM, Fiuzat M, Thompson V, Shaw LK, Neely ML, Adams KF, Whellan DJ, Donahue MP, Ahmad T, Kitzman DW, Piña IL, Zannad F, Kraus WE, O'Connor CM Soluble GPG 2 in ambulatory patients with heart failure. failure: Association with functional capacity and long-term outcomes. Circ Heart Fail. 2013 Nov; 6(6):1172-9.

96. Ahmed T, Fiuzat M, Neely B, Neely ML, Pencina MJ, Kraus WE, Zannad F, Whellan DJ, Donahue MP, Piña IL, Adams KF, Kitzman DW, O'Connor CM, Felker GM. Biomarkers of myocardial stress and fibrosis as predictors of mode of death in patients with chronic heart failure. JACC Heart Failure. 2014 Wool; 2(3):260-8.

97. Yancy CW, Jessup M, Bozkurt B, Butler J, Casey DE Jr, Colvin MM, Drazner MH, Filippatos GS, Fonarow GC, Givertz MM, Hollenberg SM, Lindenfeld

J, Masoudi FA, McBride PE, Peterson PN, Stevenson LW, Westlake C. 2017 ACC/AHA/HFCA Focused Update of the 2013 ACCF/AHA Guideline for the Management of Heart Failure: A Report of the American College of Cardiology/American Heart Association Task Force on Clinical Practice Guidelines and the Heart Failure Society of America.J Am Coll Cardiol. 2017 Aug 8; 70(6):776-803.

98. Yu Q, Watson RR, Marchalonis JJ, Larson DF. A role for T lymphocytes in mediating cardiac diastolic function. Am J Physiol Heart Circ Physiol. 2005 Aug; 289(2):H643-51.

99. Rose-John S. IL-6 trans-signaling via the soluble IL-6 receptor: importance for the pro-inflammatory activities of IL-6. Int J Biol Sci. 2012; 8(9):1237-47.

100. Fischer P, Hilfiker-Kleiner D. Survival pathways in hypertrophy and heart failure: the gp130-STAT3 axis. Basic Res Cardiol. 2007 Jul; 102(4):279-97.

101. Wasan RS, Sullivan LM, Roubenoff R, Dinarello CA, Harris T, Benjamin EJ, Sawyer DB, Levy D, Wilson PW, D'Agostino RB, Framingham Heart Study. Inflammatory markers and risk of heart failure in elderly subjects without prior myocardial infarction: the Framingham Heart Study. Circulation. 2003 Mar 25; 107(11):1486-91.

102. Yan AT, Yan RT, Cushman M, Redheuil A, Tracy RP, Arnett DK, Rosen BD, McClelland RL, Bluemke DA, Lima JA. Relationship of interleukin-6 with regional and global left-ventricular function in asymptomatic individuals without clinical cardiovascular disease: insights from the Multi-Ethnic Study of Atherosclerosis. Eur Heart J. 2010 Apr; 31(7):875-82.

103. Yokoyama T, Nakano M, Bednarczyk JL, McIntyre BW, Entman M, Mann DL. Tumor necrosis factor-alpha provokes a hypertrophic growth response in adult cardiac myocytes. Circulation. 1997 Mar 4; 95(5):1247-52.

104. Peng J, Gurantz D, Tran W, Cowling RT, Greenberg BH. Tumor necrosis factor-alpha-induced AT1 receptor upregulation enhances angiotensin II-mediated cardiac fibroblast responses that favor fibrosis. Circ Res. 2002 Dec 13; 91(12):1119-26.

105. Levine B, Kalman J, Mayer L, Fillit HM, Packer M. Elevated circulating levels of tumor necrosis factor in severe chronic heart failure. N Engl J Med. 1990 Jul 26; 323(4):236-41.

106. Miettinen KH, Lassus J, Harjola VP, Siirilä-Waris K, Melin J, Punnonen KR, Nieminen MS, Laakso M, Peuhkurinen KJ. Prognostic role of pro- and anti-inflammatory cytokines and their polymorphisms in acute decompensated heart failure. Eur J Heart Fail. 2008 Apr; 10(4):396-403.

107. Dallmeier D, Brenner H, Mons U, Rottbauer W, Koenig W, Rothenbacher D. Growth Differentiation Factor 15, Its 12-Month Relative Change, and Risk of Cardiovascular Events and Total Mortality in Patients with Stable Coronary Heart Disease: 10-Year Follow-up -up of the KAROLA Study. Clin Chem. 2016 July; 62(7):982-92.

108. Kempf T, von Haehling S, Peter T, Allhoff T, Cicoira M, Doehner W, Ponikowski P, Filippatos GS, Rosentryt P, Drexler H, Anker SD, Wollert KC. Prognostic utility of growth differentiation factor-15 in patients with chronic heart failure. J Am Coll Cardiol. 2007 Sep 11; 50(11):1054-60.

109. Anand IS, Kempf T, Rector TS, Tapken H, Allhoff T, Jantzen F, Kuskowski M, Cohn JN, Drexler H, Wollert KC. Serial measurement of growth-differentiation factor-15 in heart failure: relation to disease severity and prognosis in the Valsartan Heart Failure Trial. Circulation. 2010 Oct 5; 122(14):1387-95.

110. Kawanabe Y, Nauli SM. Endothelin. Cell Mol Life Sci. 2011 Jean; 68(2):195-203.

111. Hülsmann M, Stanek B, Frey B, Sturm B, Putz D, Kos T, Berger R, Woloszczuk W, Putz D, Kos T, Berger R, Woloszczuk W, Maurer G, Pacher R. Value of cardiopulmonary exercise testing and large endothelin plasma levels to predict short-term prognosis of patients with chronic heart failure. J Am Coll Cardiol. 1998 Nov 15; 32(6):1695-700.

112. O'Seaghdha CM, Hwang SJ, Ho JE, Wasan RS, Levy D, Fox CS. Elevated galectin-3 precedes the development of CKD. J Am Soc Nephrol. 2013;24(9):1470-1477.

113. Uren NG, Melin JA, De Bruyne B, Wijns W, Baudhuin T, Camici PG. Relationship between myocardial blood flow and the severity of coronary artery stenosis. N Engl J Med, 330 (1994), pp. 1782-8.

114. Neishi, Y., Akasaka, T., Tsukiji, M., Kume, T., Wada, N., Watanabe, N., Kawamoto, T., Kaji, S., & Yoshida, K. (2005). Reduced coronary flow reserve in patients with congestive heart failure assessed by transthoracic Doppler echocardiography. Journal of the American Society of Echocardiography : official publication of the American Society of Echocardiography, 18(1), 15–19.

115. Rigo F, Gherardi S, Galderisi M, Sicari R, Picano E. The independent prognostic value of contractile and coronary flow reserve determined by dipyridamole stress echocardiography in patients with idiopathic dilated cardiomyopathy. Am J Cardiol. 2007 Apr 15; 99(8):1154-8.

116. Rigo F, Gherardi S, Galderisi M, Pratali L, Cortigiani L, Sicari R, Picano E. The prognostic impact of coronary flow-reserve assessed by Doppler echocardiography in non-ischaemic dilated cardiomyopathy. Eur Heart J. 2006 Wool; 27(11):1319-23.

117. Folse R, Braunwald E (1962) Determination of fraction of left ventricular volume ejected per beat and of ventricular end-diastolic and residual volumes. Experimental and clinical observations with a precordial dilution technique. Circulation 25:674–685.

118. Bartle SH, Sanmarco ME, Dammann JF Jr (1965) Ejected fraction: an index of myocardial function. Am J Cardiol 15(1):125.

119. Jhund PS & McMurray JJV. The neprilysin pathway in heart failure: a review and guide on the use of sacubitril/valsartan. Heart 2016;102(17):1342–1347.

120. Mebazaa A et al. Acute heart failure and cardiogenic shock: a multidisciplinary practical guidance. Intensive Care Med. 42, 147–163 (2015).

121. Fudim M et al. Aetiology, timing and clinical predictors of early vs. late readmission following index hospitalization for acute heart failure: insights from ASCEND-HF. Eur. J. Heart Fail. 20, 304–314 (2018).

122. Braunwald E, Kloner RA. The stunned myocardium: prolonged,

postischemic ventricular dysfunction. Circulation. 1982; 66:1146–1149.

123. Guaricci AI, Bulzis G, Pontone G, Scicchitano P, Carbonara R, Rabbat M, De Santis D, Ciccone MM. Current interpretation of myocardial stunning. Trends Cardiovasc Med. 2018; 28:263–27.

124. Wdowiak-Okrojek K, Wejner-Mik P, Kasprzak JD, Lipiec P. Recovery of regional systolic and diastolic myocardial function after acute myocardial infarction evaluated by two-dimensional speckle tracking echocardiography. Clin Physiol Funct Imaging. 2019; 39:177–181.

125. Maranta F, Tondi L, Agricola E, Margonato A, Rimoldi O, Camici PG. Ivabradine reduces myocardial stunning in patients with exercise-inducible ischemia. Basic Res Cardiol. 2015; 110:55.

126. Kubo SH, Rector TS, Bank AJ, Williams RE, Heifetz SM. Endothelium-dependent vasodilation is attenuated in patients with heart failure. Circulation. 1991 Oct; 84(4):1589-96.

127. Guazzi M, Samaja M, Arena R, Vicenzi M, Guazzi MD. Long-term use of sildenafil in the therapeutic management of heart failure. J Am Coll Cardiol. 2007 Nov 27; 50(22):2136-44.

128. Borlaug BA, Melenovsky V, Russell SD, Kessler K, Pacak K, Becker LC, Kass DA. Impaired chronotropic and vasodilator reserves limit exercise capacity in patients with heart failure and a preserved ejection fraction. Circulation. 2006 Nov 14; 114(20):2138-47.

129. van Empel VP, Mariani J, Borlaug BA, Kaye DM. Impaired myocardial oxygen availability contributes to abnormal exercise hemodynamics in heart failure with preserved ejection fraction. J Am Heart Assoc. 2014 Dec 2; 3(6):e001293.

130. Borlaug BA, Kane GC, Melenovsky V, Olson TP. Abnormal right ventricular-pulmonary artery coupling with exercise in heart failure with preserved ejection fraction. Eur Heart J. 2016 Nov 14; 37(43):3293-3302.

131. Paulus WJ, Tschöpe C. A novel paradigm for heart failure with preserved ejection fraction: comorbidities drive myocardial dysfunction and remodeling through coronary microvascular endothelial inflammation. J Am Coll Cardiol. 2013

Jul 23; 62(4):263-71.

132. Mohammed SF, Hussain S, Mirzoyev SA, Edwards WD, Maleszewski JJ, Redfield MM. Coronary microvascular rarefaction and myocardial fibrosis in heart failure with preserved ejection fraction. Circulation. 2015 Feb 10; 131(6):550-9.

133. Borlaug BA, Melenovsky V, Russell SD, Kessler K, Pacak K, Becker LC, Kass DA. Impaired chronotropic and vasodilator reserves limit exercise capacity in patients with heart failure and a preserved ejection fraction. Circulation. 2006 Nov 14; 114(20):2138-47.

134. DorFC S, Zeh W, Hochholzer W, Jander N, Kienzle RP, Pieske B, Neumann FJ. Pulmonary capillary wedge pressure during exercise and long-term mortality in patients with suspected heart failure with preserved ejection fraction. Eur Heart J. 2014 Nov 21; 35(44):3103-12.

135. Mosterd A, Hoes AW. Clinical epidemiology of heart failure. Heart 2007;93:1137–46. doi:10.1136/hrt.2003.025270

136. Roger VL: Epidemiology of heart failure. Circ Res 2013; 113: pp. 646-659.

137. Role of renal sympathetic nerves in mediating hypoperfusion of renal cortical microcirculation in experimental congestive heart failure and acute extracellular fluid volume depletion. J Clin Invest 76:1913–1920, 1985.

138. Ramchandra R, Hood SG, Frithiof R, May CN. Discharge properties of cardiac and renal sympathetic nerves and their impaired responses to changes in blood volume in heart failure. Am J PhysiolRegulIntegr Comp Physiol 297: R665–R674, 2009.

139. DiBona GF, Sawin LL. Role of renal alpha 2-adrenergic receptors in spontaneously hypertensive rats. Hypertension 9:41–48, 1987.

140. Bergdahl A, Valdemarsson S, Pantev E, Ottosson A, Feng QP, Sun XY, Hedner T, Edvinsson L. Modulation of vascular contractile responses to alpha 1- and alpha 2-adrenergic and neuropeptide Y receptor stimulation in rats with ischemic heart failure. Acta PhysiolScand 154: 429–437, 1995.

141. Teerlink JR, Gray GA, Clozel M, Clozel JP. Increased vascular responsiveness to norepinephrine in rats with heart failure is endothelium dependent.

Dissociation of basal and stimulated nitric oxide release. Circulation 89:393–401, 1994.

142. F. Triposkiadis, G. Karayannis, G. Giamouzis, J. Skoularigis, G. Louridas, J. Butler The sympathetic nervous system in heart failure: physiology, pathophysiology, and clinical implications J Am Coll Cardiol, 54 (2009), pp. 1747-1762.

143. PJ Schwartz Vagal stimulation for heart disease: from animals to men Circ J, 75 (2011), pp. 20-27.

144. PJ Schwarts, GM Ferrari Sympathetic-parasympathetic interaction in health and disease: abnormalities and relevance in heart failure Heart Fail Rev, 16 (2011), pp. 101-107.

145. Chaggar PS, Malkin CJ, Shaw SM, et al. Neuroendocrine effects on the heart and targets for therapeutic manipulation in heart failure. Cardiovasc Ther2009;27:187–93.

146. McMurray JJ, Packer M, Desai AS, et al. Angiotensin-neprilysin inhibition versus enalapril in heart failure. N Engl J Med 2014;371:993–1004.

147. Milliez P, Girerd H, Plouin PF, Blacher J, Safar ME, Mourad JJ. Evidence for an increased rate of cardiovascular events in patients with primary aldosteronism. Journal of the American College of Cardiology. 2005;45(8):1243-1248.

148. Munzel T, Gori T, Keaney JF Jr, Maack C, Daiber A. Pathophysiological role of oxidative stress in systolic and diastolic heart failure and its therapeutic implications. European Heart Journal. 2015;36(38):2555-2564.

149. Ponikowski P, Voors AA, Anker SD, Bueno H, Cleland JG, Coats AJ, Falk V, González-Juanatey JR, Harjola VP, Jankowska EA, Jessup M, Linde C, Nihoyannopoulos P, Parissis JT, Pieske B, Riley JP, Rosano GM, Ruilope LM, Ruschitzka F, Rutten FH, van der Meer P. 2016 ESC Guidelines for the diagnosis and treatment of acute and chronic heart failure: The Task Force for the diagnosis and treatment of acute and chronic heart failure of the European Society of Cardiology (ESC). Developed with the special contribution of the Heart Failure Association (HFA) of the ESC. Eur J Heart Fail 2016;18:891–975.

150. Levin ER, Gardner DG, Samson WK. Natriuretic peptides. N Engl J Med 1998;339:321–328.

151. Calvieri C, Rubattu S, Volpe M. Molecular mechanisms underlying cardiac antihypertrophic and antifibrotic effects of natriuretic peptides. J Mol Med (Berl) 2012;90:5–13.

152. Flather MD, Yusuf S, Køber L, Pfeffer M, Hall A, Murray G, Torp-Pedersen C, Ball S, Pogue J, Moyé L, Braunwald E. Long-term ACE-inhibitor therapy in patients with heart failure or left- ventricular dysfunction: a systematic overview of data from individual patients. ACE-Inhibitor Myocardial Infarction Collaborative Group. Lancet. 2000 May 6; 355(9215):1575-81.

153. Bristow MR, Gilbert EM, Abraham WT, Adams KF, Fowler MB, Hershberger RE, Kubo SH, Narahara KA, Ingersoll H, Krueger S, Young S, Shusterman N. Carvedilol produces dose-related improvements in left ventricular function and survival in subjects with chronic heart failure. MOCHA Investigators. Circulation. 1996 Dec 1; 94(11):2807-16.

154. Pitt B, Pedro Ferreira J, Zannad F. Mineralocorticoid receptor antagonists in patients with heart failure: current experience and future perspectives. Eur Heart J Cardiovasc Pharmacother. 2017 Jan; 3(1):48-57.

155. McMurray JJ, Ostergren J, Swedberg K, Granger CB, Held P, Michelson EL, OloFCson B, Yusuf S, Pfeffer MA, CHARM Investigators and Committees. Effects of candesartan in patients with chronic heart failure and reduced left-ventricular systolic function taking angiotensin-converting-enzyme inhibitors: the CHARM-Added trial. Lancet. 2003 Sep 6; 362(9386):767-71.

156. Choi KH, Lee GY, Choi JO, Jeon ES, Lee HY, Lee SE, Kim JJ, Chae SC, Baek SH, Kang SM, Choi DJ, Yoo BS, Kim KH, Cho MC, Park HY, Oh BH. The mortality benefit of carvedilol versus bisoprolol in patients with heart failure with reduced ejection fraction. Korean J Intern Med. 2019 Sep; 34(5):1030-1039.

157. Swedberg K, Komajda M, Bohm M, et al. Ivabradine and outcomes in chronic heart failure (SHIFT): a randomized placebo-controlled study. Lancet. 2010;376:875–885.

158. Felker GM, Mentz RJ, Adams KF, Cole RT, Egnaczyk GF, Patel CB, Fiuzat M, Gregory D, Wedge P, O'Connor CM, Udelson JE, Konstam MA. Tolvaptan in Patients Hospitalized With Acute Heart Failure: Rationale and Design of the TACTICS and SECRET of CHF Trials. Circ Heart Fail. 2015 Sep; 8(5):997-1005.

159. Lytvyn Y, Bjornstad P, Udell JA, Lovshin JA, Cherney DZI. Sodium Glucose Cotransporter-2 Inhibition in Heart Failure: Potential Mechanisms, Clinical Applications, and Summary of Clinical Trials. Circulation. 2017 Oct 24; 136(17):1643-1658.

160. Neal B, Perkovic V, Mahaffey KW, et al. Canagliflozin and cardiovascular and renal events in type 2 diabetes. N Engl J Med. 2017;377:644–657.

161. Marceau SP, Daniels GH, Brown-Frandsen K, et al. Liraglutide and cardiovascular outcomes in type 2 diabetes. N Engl J Med. 2016;375:311–322.

162. Results of the Cooperative North Scandinavian Enalapril Survival Study (CONSENSUS). CONSENSUS Trial Study Group. Effects of enalapril on mortality in severe congestive heart failure. N Engl J Med. 1987 Jun 4; 316(23):1429-35.

163. SOLVD Investigators., Yusuf S, Pitt B, Davis CE, Hood WB, Cohn JN Effect of enalapril on survival in patients with reduced left ventricular ejection fraction and congestive heart failure. N Engl J Med. 1991 Aug 1; 325(5):293-302.

164. Packer M, Poole-Wilson PA, Armstrong PW, Cleland JG, Horowitz JD, Massie BM, Rydén L, Thygesen K, Uretsky BF. Comparative effects of low and high doses of the angiotensin-converting enzyme inhibitor, lisinopril, on morbidity and mortality in chronic heart failure. ATLAS Study Group. Circulation. 1999 Dec 7; 100(23):2312-8.

165. Cleland JG, Tendera M, Adamus J, Freemantle N, Polonski L, Taylor J, PEP-CHF Investigators. The perindopril in elderly people with chronic heart failure (PEP-CHF) study. Eur Heart J. 2006 Oct; 27(19):2338-45.

166. Jin Joo Park, Alexandre Mebazaa, In Chang Hwang, Jun Bean Park, Jae Hyeong Park et al. Phenotyping Heart Failure According to Longitudinal Ejection Fraction Change: Myocardial Strain, Predictors, and Outcomes Journal of the American Heart Association. 2020;9:e015009.

167. Fonarow GC, Abraham WT, Albert NM, et al. Organized Program to Initiate Lifesaving Treatment in Hospitalized Patients with Heart Failure

(OPTIMIZE-HF): rationale and design. Am Heart J. 2004;148(1):43-51. doi:10.1016/j.ahj.2004.03.004

168. oung JB, Dunlap ME, Pfeffer MA, et al. Mortality and morbidity reduction with Candesartan in patients with chronic heart failure and left ventricular systolic dysfunction: results of the CHARM low-left ventricular ejection fraction trials. Circulation. 2004;110(17):2618-2626. doi:10.1161/01.CIR.0000146819.43235.A9

169. Oscalices MIL, Okuno MFP, Lopez MCBT, Batista REA, Campanharo CRV. Health literacy and adherence to treatment of patients with heart failure. Rev Esc Enferm USP. 2019;53:e03447. Published 2019 Jul 15. doi:10.1590/S1980-220X2017039803447

170. Paolillo S, Scardovi AB, Campodonico J. Role of comorbidities in heart failure prognosis Part I: Anemia, iron deficiency, diabetes, atrial fibrillation. Eur J PrevCardiol. 2020;27(2_suppl):27-34. doi:10.1177/2047487320960288

171. Špinar J, Špinarová L, Vítovec J. Pathophysiology, causes and epidemiology of chronic heart failure. Patofiziologie, cause epidemiologiechronickéhosredčníhoselhání. Vnitr Lek. 2018;64(9):834-838.

172. Brennan EJ. Chronic heart failure nursing: integrated multidisciplinary care. Br J Nurs. 2018;27(12):681-688. doi:10.12968/bjon.2018.27.12.681

173. Witte KK, Clark AL. Why does chronic heart failure cause breathlessness and fatigue? Prog Cardiovasc Dis. 2007;49(5):366-384. doi:10.1016/j.pcad.2006.10.003

174. King M, Kingery J, Casey B. Diagnosis and evaluation of heart failure. Am Fam Physician. 2012;85(12):1161-1168.

175. Chen YW, Wang CY, Lai YH, et al. Home-based cardiac rehabilitation improves quality of life, aerobic capacity, and readmission rates in patients with chronic heart failure. Medicine (Baltimore). 2018;97(4):e9629. doi:10.1097/MD.0000000000009629

176. Taylor RS, Walker S, Ciani O, et al. Exercise-based cardiac rehabilitation for chronic heart failure: the EXTRAMATCH II individual participant data meta-analysis. Health Technol Assess. 2019;23(25):1-98. doi:10.3310/hta23250

177. Du H, Wonggom P, Tongpeth J, Clark RA. Six-Minute Walk Test for Assessing Physical Functional Capacity in Chronic Heart Failure. Curr Heart Fail

Rep. 2017;14(3):158-166. doi:10.1007/s11897-017-0330-3

178. Pinho-Gomes AC, Rahimi K. Management of blood pressure in heart failure. Heart. 2019;105(8):589-595. doi:10.1136/heartjnl-2018-314438

179. Nikolovska Vukadinović A, Vukadinović D, Borer J, et al. Heart rate and its reduction in chronic heart failure and beyond. Eur J Heart Fail. 2017;19(10):1230-1241. doi:10.1002/ejhf.902

180. Kowalczys A, Bohdan M, Gruchała M. Prognostic value of daytime heart rate, blood pressure, their products and quotients in chronic heart failure. Cardiol J. 2019;26(1):20-28. doi:10.5603/CJ.a2017.0130

181. Böhm M, Young R, Jhund PS, et al. Systolic blood pressure, cardiovascular outcomes and efficacy and safety of sacubitril/valsartan (LCZ696) in patients with chronic heart failure and reduced ejection fraction: results from PARADIGM-HF. Eur Heart J. 2017;38(15):1132-1143. doi:10.1093/eurheartj/ehw570

182. Del Buono MG, Mihalick V, Damonte JI, et al. Preservation of Cardiac Reserve and Cardiorespiratory Fitness in Patients With Acute De Novo Versus Acute on Chronic Heart Failure With Reduced Ejection Fraction. Am J Cardiol. 2021;158:74-80. doi:10.1016/j.amjcard.2021.07.036

183. Richer C, Domergue V, Gervais M, Fornes P, Trabold F, Giudicelli JF. Coronary dilatation reserve in experimental hypertension and chronic heart failure: effects of blockade of the renin-angiotensin system. Clin Exp Pharmacol Physiol. 2001;28(12):997-1001. doi:10.1046/j.1440-1681.2001.03573.x

184. Rørth R, Jhund PS, Yilmaz MB, et al. Comparison of BNP and NT-proBNP in Patients With Heart Failure and Reduced Ejection Fraction. Circ Heart Fail. 2020;13(2):e006541.doi:10.1161/CIRCHEARTFAILURE.119.006541

185. Pontremoli R, Borghi C, Perrone Filardi P. Renal protection in chronic heart failure: focus on sacubitril/valsartan. Eur Heart J Cardiovasc Pharmacother. 2021;7(5):445-452. doi:10.1093/ehjcvp/pvab030

# LIST OF CONVENTIONS AND ABBREVIATIONS

ACEI is an angiotensin-converting enzyme inhibitor

AB - arterial pressure

AST - aspartate aminotransferase

ACS - aortic coronary bypass

ALT - alanine aminotransferase

ARB is an angiotensin receptor blocker

BB is a beta blocker

BMQAO'B - an acute disorder of blood circulation in the brain

DBP - diastolic arterial blood pressure

Ж is the size of the coin

FC - functional class

QD - diabetes mellitus

PKA - right carotid artery

PNA - anterior descending artery

SABP - systolic arterial blood pressure

CRP – C-reactive protein

CHF - chronic heart failure

SBK is a chronic kidney disease

TAZ - coronary artery reserve volume

TMI - body mass index

COPD is a chronic obstructive lung disease

ED – endothelial dysfunction

OF - firing fraction

EFCHF - heart failure observed with a decrease in ejection fraction

OFCCHF - heart failure with preserved ejection fraction

AEFCHF - heart failure with a slightly reduced or borderline ejection fraction

CHD is an ischemic heart disease

HIGH is the number of heart contractions

ChB – left lobe

ChQ - left ventricle

ChQ SDO' is the end-diastolic size of the left ventricle

ChQ SDH – left ventricular end-diastolic volume

ChQ SSO' is the end-systolic size of the left ventricle

ChQ SSH is the end-systolic volume of the left ventricle

ChQG - left ventricular hypertrophy

MRA is a mineralocorticoid receptor antagonist

BNP - brain natriuretic protein

NT-proBNP – N-terminal brain natriuretic protein

NYHA – New York Heart Association

TAPSE - Estimation of Tricuspid Valve Systolic Excursion

Vpd – peak blood flow velocity (pressure) in diastole

# TABLE OF CONTENTS

**Abstract**..................................................................................

1.1. Epidemiology and prevalence of chronic heart failure..............................................................................

1.2. Clinical presentation and classification of chronic heart failure..............................................................................
...............

1.3. Modern pathophysiological mechanisms of the development of chronic heart failure..............................................................

1.4. Importance of modern biomarkers in chronic heart failure.
..............................................

1.5. Cardiovascular functional status in chronic heart failure..............................................................................
..................

1.6. Blocking various neurohumoral control systems in chronic heart failure..............................................................

1.7. Modern approaches to the pharmacological treatment of chronic heart failure..............................................................................

**Precipitating factors of chronic heart failure decompensation**................................................................

• 2.1. Characterization of patients in the study according to left ventricular ejection fraction and phenotypic groups of the disease.

2.1.1. Clinical demographic characteristics of patients..................

2.1.2. Precipitating factors of chronic heart failure decompensation...................................... ............................................

2.1.3. Clinical and hemodynamic parameters of the patients included in the investigation according to the ejection fraction............................................... ...

2.1.4. Results of laboratory tests................................................ ...

2.1.5. Prehospital treatment of chronic heart failure

2.1.6. Evaluation of central hemodynamic indicators, myocardial condition and reserve of coronary arteries............................................... ...........

• 2.2. Assessment of the activity of the sodium-uretic peptide system and the structural and functional state of the myocardium in patients with CHF.

# EVALUATION OF THE EFFICACY OF 12 WEEKS OF SACUBITRIL/VALSARTAN TREATMENT ON PATIENT CLINICAL AND FUNCTIONAL STATUS................................. ....

• 3.1. Clinical demographic indicators of patients................................

• 3.2. Initial clinical and hemodynamic parameters of patients in groups.................................... ............................................. ....

• 3.3. Initial laboratory test indicators of patients in groups.................................. ........................................... ...

3.3.1. Pre-hospital treatment of patients in groups................

3.3.2. Indicators of initial coronary reserve and myocardial condition of patients in groups............................................. ..

• 3.4. Efficacy, safety, and effects on clinical and biochemical parameters of 12-week treatment with sacubitril/valsartan. ...............................................

• 3.5. Effects of 12-week treatment with sacubitril/valsartan on central and peripheral hemodynamic parameters, myocardial reserve volume and viability. ......................

**TERMINATIONS**..............................................

..........................................

**LIST OF REFERENCES**...............................
**LIST OF CONVENTIONS AND ABBREVIATIONS**.................

www.ingramcontent.com/pod-product-compliance
Lightning Source LLC
LaVergne TN
LVHW080354070526
838199LV00059B/3807